# Group Therapy for Psychoses

T0141237

Group therapy for patients with psychotic experiences is one of the least known of the group therapies; but it is also one of the most diverse. This collection presents a range of methods, models and settings for group therapy for psychoses, as well as exploring the context for this type of treatment.

*Group Therapy for Psychoses* offers an international perspective on the current range of practice in the field, and in multiple care situations, contexts and institutions: from acute units to therapeutic communities, rehabilitation groups, self-help, and groups of those who hear voices. Presented in two parts, the first covers the history, evaluation and research methodologies of group therapy, while the second part explores specific examples of groups and settings. This book tackles misconceptions about the treatment of psychoses and emphasises the healing effects of group therapy. It underscores the importance of training for selecting and conducting groups of patients suffering from psychoses, and suggests possible formats, approaches and perspectives.

This book's wide, reflective and practical collection of chapters together demonstrate how group therapies can effectively help patients with psychotic experiences to overcome their difficulties on their way to recovery. The book will be of great use to clinicians working with people suffering from psychosis, including psychiatrists, psychotherapists, psychoanalysts, psychologists, physicians and social workers. It will also appeal to group analysts, family therapists and cognitive behavioural therapy practitioners, as well as to researchers in all these fields.

**Ivan Urlić** is a neuropsychiatrist, psychoanalytic psychotherapist, group analyst and Professor of Psychiatry and Psychological Medicine at the Medical School, University of Split, Croatia. He is a founder member of the Institute of Group Analysis (IGA) Zagreb and IGA Bologna, where he is a training group analyst and supervisor.

**Manuel González de Chávez** is the former President of the ISPS (International Society for Psychological and Social Approaches to Psychosis). He is currently the President of the Foundation for Research and Treatment of Schizophrenia in Madrid, Spain. Until his retirement, he was Head of the Psychiatry Service at the Hospital General Universitario Gregorio Marañón of Madrid and Professor of Psychiatry at the Complutense University of Madrid. He was also Director of Mental Health Services in Seville, President of the Mental Health Association of Madrid and President of the Spanish Association of Neuropsychiatry.

# Group Therapy for Psychoses

*Edited by*
Ivan Urlić and
Manuel González de Chávez

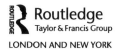
Routledge
Taylor & Francis Group

LONDON AND NEW YORK

First published 2019
by Routledge
2 Park Square, Milton Park, Abingdon, Oxon OX14 4RN

and by Routledge
711 Third Avenue, New York, NY 10017

*Routledge is an imprint of the Taylor & Francis Group, an informa business*

*British Library Cataloguing in Publication Data*
A catalogue record for this book is available from the British Library

*Library of Congress Cataloging in Publication Data*
Names: Urlić, Ivan, editor. | González de Chávez, Manuel, editor.
Title: Group therapy for psychoses / [edited by] Ivan Urlić and
Manuel González de Chávez.
Description: Abingdon, Oxon ; New York, NY : Routledge, 2019. |
Includes bibliographical references.
Identifiers: LCCN 2018013024 (print) | LCCN 2018015788 (ebook) |
ISBN 9781315522616 (Master e-book) | ISBN 9781138697096
(hardback) | ISBN 9781138697102 (pbk.) | ISBN 9781315522616 (ebk)
Subjects: | MESH: Psychotic Disorders—therapy | Psychotherapy, Group
Classification: LCC RC480.5 (ebook) | LCC RC480.5 (print) |
NLM WM 200 | DDC 616.89/14—dc23
LC record available at https://lccn.loc.gov/2018013024

ISBN: 978-1-138-69709-6 (hbk)
ISBN: 978-1-138-69710-2 (pbk)
ISBN: 978-1-315-52261-6 (ebk)

Typeset in Times New Roman
by Keystroke, Neville Lodge, Tettenhall, Wolverhampton

# Contents

## PART II
## Groups for psychoses: Different approaches and
## different settings                                                    39

# Notes on contributors

**Bojana Avguštin Avčin, MD, Ph.D.,** is a psychiatrist and group analyst. She works as a consultant psychiatrist at the University psychiatric hospital in Ljubljana. Her special interests concern the use of group setting in the psychotherapy of patients with psychosis, and she has published several papers on this topic. She is also an active participant in many international professional events, being a member of the Slovenian Medical Association, ISPS International and Slovenia, and Group Analytic Society of Slovenia.

**Chyrell Bellamy, M.S.W., Ph.D.,** is an Assistant Professor of Psychiatry at the Yale School of Medicine, where she serves as the Director of Peer Services and Research at the Program for Recovery and Community Health. She has experience as a frontline service provider, community educator and organiser, instructor in psychology and social work, community and academic researcher, and as a person in recovery. Her expertise includes developing and conducting community-based research initiatives in partnership with people with lived experience. Her research examines: sociocultural pathways of recovery from mental illness, with a particular focus on health disparities; research and practice experience in the area of peer-support services; group-work interventions; spirituality; health promotion; and culture and recovery.

**Marjeta Blinc Pesek, MD, MSc,** is a psychiatrist and group analyst in private practice. She is a member of the Slovenian Medical Association, the European psychiatric association, ISPS International, President of ISPS Slovenia from 2005, and Secretary of Group Analytic Society of Slovenia from 2011. She is organiser of the Slovenian ISPS Annual Workshop. She has published many papers regarding the psychological/psychodynamic approach to patients with psychosis and their families, especially in group settings. For her professional activities, she was awarded with the Prešern Prize for student research from the University of Ljubljana.

**Anamarija Bogović Dijaković** is a clincal pychologist at the Sestre Milosrdnice, University Hospital Centre, in Zagreb. She is also Assistant Professor in the Department of Psychology at the Catholic University of Croatia. Already trained in cognitive behavioural therapy, she is currently training in group analysis. Her research interests include psychiatric disorders and their features, as well as psychological assessment and counselling.

**Larry Davidson, Ph.D.,** is a Professor of Psychiatry at the Yale School of Medicine, where he directs the Program for Recovery and Community Health. He also serves as the Chief Policy Advisor for the Connecticut Department of Mental Health and Addiction Services. His research has focused on processes of recovery in serious mental illnesses and addictions, and the development, evaluation and dissemination of social policies and innovative community-based programmes to promote recovery and community inclusion among persons with these conditions.

**Margreet de Pater** is a community psychiatrist. She developed Transmural Family Guidance after having worked in the Crisis Centre Utrecht and in the Multifunctional Unit in Altrecht. Her book, *The Loneliness of Psychosis*, will soon be translated into English.

**Simone Donnari** is an art therapist who developed an innovative video-integration method in the field of art therapy. Together with Maurizio Peciccia, he developed an original method for the therapy of psychoses, called 'amniotic therapy'. He is Educational Director at Art Therapy School of Assisi and he is co-founder of Istituto Gaetano Benedetti, school of psychotherapy. He is Vice President of the Italian professional association of art therapists (APIArt). In 1995, he co-founded Sementera Onlus, the association dedicated to therapeutic activities for the social rehabilitation of psychotic and autistic patients. In 2011, he co-founded ISPS Italy. Since 2013, he is co-Head of the research project 'Bodily self and social interaction: Sensorimotor and autonomic correlated and motor sensory integration therapies in chronic schizophrenic patients'. He regularly performs seminars, lectures and supervisory sessions in mental health centres in Italy, the University of Perugia and New York University Steinhardt.

**Maria Edwards** is the Director of Peer Services at the Connecticut Mental Health Center of the Department of Psychiatry at the Yale School of Medicine. She co-leads a home group.

**Ruth Firmin** is a doctoral student at Purdue University, Indianapolis, studying clinical psychology. She is currently a Psychology Fellow in the Yale School of Medicine, Department of Psychiatry, working in community mental health, where she has had the opportunity to co-lead groups with peer providers. Her research examines factors that impact recovery, particularly stigma and stigma resistance.

**Ignacio García Cabeza** is a psychiatrist at the University Hospital Gregorio Marañón and Associate Professor in the Complutense University of Madrid. He also coordinates ISPS Spain. Actively involved in developing psychotherapeutically oriented programmes for psychotic patients, his focus is mainly on group psychotherapeutic interventions. He has collaborated in the organisation of several national and international activities, including the 16th International Congress of the ISPS (member of the Organizing and Scientific Committee), and the Annual Course of Schizophrenia, the most popular course about psychosis in Spain. He has published research in journals such as: *Schizophrenia Research*, *Acta Psychiatrica Scandinavica*, *European Psychiatry*, *Psychosis* and *Group Analysis*.

**Manuel González de Chávez** is ex-President of the ISPS and is currently President of the Foundation for Research and Treatment of Schizophrenia and Other Psychoses, as well as organising the Annual Course of Schizophrenia in Madrid. For about 20 years, until his recent retirement, he was Chief of the Psychiatry Service 1 at the Hospital General Universitario Gregorio Marañón, and Professor of Psychiatry at the Complutense University of Madrid. He was also Director of the Mental Health Services of Seville, President of the Mental Health Association of Madrid, and President of the Spanish Association of Neuropsychiatry, of which he is an Honorary Member. Dedicated to the development of psychotherapeutic programmes for psychotic patients, and especially to group psychotherapy in schizophrenia and its importance in the treatment of these patients, he is author and editor of several books and many publications on this subject.

**Majda Grah, Ph.D.,** graduated from the School of Medicine, University of Zagreb, Croatia, in 1993. She is a psychiatrist, psychotherapist, group analyst and supervisor in group analysis. At the psychiatric hospital Sveti Ivan in Zagreb, she is Head of the psychotherapeutic department for the treatment of affective, anxious, dissociative, and personality disorders, where she conducts psychotherapeutic groups for neurotic, psychotic and patients with personality disorders. The author of many articles from a group psychotherapy/analysis perspective, her professional interests concern early intervention in the first episode of psychosis, as well as programmes for the treatment of borderline personality disorders.

**Sheila Grandison** is an art psychotherapist with over 20 years' experience working in both acute and community NHS adult mental health settings. She is currently Lead Art Psychotherapist and Head of Arts Therapies in the Newham Directorate of the East London NHS Foundation Trust. She holds an Honorary Lectureship in the School of Health Sciences, City University, London, and is a past Chairperson of the British Association of Art Therapists and a founder member of ISPS UK. Since 2008, she has worked in partnership with Community Learning, Tate Modern, on projects related to social justice, mental health and art. She is co-editor of the ISPS book *Experiences of Mental Health*.

**Cecilio Hernández,** a graduate in medicine and surgery (La Laguna University, Tenerife, Spain, 1983), has specialised in psychiatry. He has worked in the

Psychiatric Hospital of Tenerife and, since 2011, in the Assertive Community Treatment Team (ECA) of the Spanish National Health System. As Head of the ECA team, he has organised different individual and group therapies for patients with schizophrenia. He has published several papers on psychiatry in regards to the rehabilitation of schizophrenic patients. Recently, he has co-authored an evaluation report on health technologies of the Spanish National Health System on group psychotherapy for persons with schizophrenia.

**Val Jackson, MSc,** is a qualified occupational therapist and systemic psychotherapist, mostly working in adult mental health services. She has run numerous therapeutic groups, especially those involving families, both with the Carers Service, and with the acute admission ward. Since 2011, she has run multi-family workshops, as well as being involved in staff training and lecturing. Her current interests include organising a trial in Open Dialogue, with the associated training workshops and special interest groups.

**David Kennard** is a clinical psychologist and group analyst. He has worked in therapeutic communities for acute psychiatric admissions and for drug addiction, both in a high security hospital, and in outpatient psychotherapy and counselling centres. While Head of Psychology at The Retreat, York, he helped to develop psychosis rehabilitation services. He has had a long involvement in the development of therapeutic communities in the UK and has published widely in the field, including *An Introduction to Therapeutic Communities* (1983, 1998). From 1992 to 1998 he was editor of the journal *Therapeutic Communities*. He has also been Chair of ISPS UK. Since retiring in 2004, he has continued to write, teach and supervise.

**Anastassios E. Koukis, Ph.D., BSc,** is a psychologist, group analyst and psychoanalyst. He is a full member of Group Analytic Society International (GASi, London) and a member of the International Association for Group Psychotherapy and Group Processes (IAGP). He is also founder and current President of ISPS Hellas. He is the author of the book *Dreams in Group Analysis* (2004) and has published many papers on group analysis, especially on the group psychotherapy of psychoses. He is involved in professional activities internationally.

**Tania Lecomte, Ph.D.,** is Professor of Psychology at the Université de Montréal and a registered clinical psychologist. She has developed and validated assessment tools and group interventions for individuals with severe mental illness, including; self-esteem enhancement groups, CBT for psychosis, CBT for parents of individuals with psychosis, CBT for supported employment, as well as mindfulness, acceptance and compassion groups. Some of these interventions are now being used across the globe. She has published many papers, as well as being the author of *Group CBT for Psychosis – A clinician's guide* (2016).

**Ana Magerle, MD,** is a psychiatrist, forensic psychiatrist and group analyst. For the last 27 years, she has been Head of the Department of Forensics in the psychiatric hospital Dr. Ivan Barbot in Popovača, Croatia. Her professional interests include inpatient and outpatient group psychotherapy on psychotic patients and severely disturbed patients. She is the author of several professional papers and book chapters.

**Susan Mao** is a doctoral candidate in the Counseling Psychology Ph.D. programme at Teachers College, Columbia University, and is currently a Psychology Fellow in the Yale University Department of Psychiatry at the Connecticut Mental Health Center (CMHC). Her research focuses on the mental health impacts of oppression, provider multicultural competence, and community-based approaches to research, practice and training. In her clinical work, she utilises integrative strengths-based and person-centered approaches with individuals on their journeys of recovery. As a Fellow at CMHC, she is currently co-facilitating a home group with a peer provider.

**Nina Mayer** graduated from the School of Medicine, University of Zagreb, Croatia, in 1996. She is a psychiatrist, psychotherapist and group analyst. Working in the psychiatric hospital Sveti Ivan in Zagreb, in the department for early interventions in psychotic disorders, she is involved with inpatient and outpatient groups for people with psychotic experiences, from acute episodes to chronic psychoses (schizophrenia). She is now completing her doctoral studies and has written papers concerning group psychotherapy for persons with psychosis, and early interventions in psychotic disorders.

**Kaja Medved, BA,** is a graduate psychologist and a consultant psychotherapist on the Crisis phoneline. She is a member of the Slovenian Psychological Association, ISPS International and Slovenia, and Group Analytic Society of Slovenia.

**Nataša Orešković-Krezler, MD,** is a psychiatrist and group analyst. She has been practising group psychotherapy in inpatient and outpatient settings for the two largest psychiatric hospitals in Croatia for 20 years. For the last 15 years, she has worked in private practice in Zagreb. Her fields of interest are psychotherapy of severely disturbed patients, borderline and PTSD patients, and especially psychotic patients in group-analytic settings. She is the author of several professional papers.

**Anthony J. Pavlo, Ph.D.,** is an Associate Research Scientist at the Yale University Program for Recovery and Community Health. He completed his doctoral studies in clinical psychology at Miami University and his graduate research investigated a person-centered alternative to psychiatric diagnosis. His current research interests include healthcare relationships, person-centered practices, and recovery-oriented approaches to care.

**Maurizio Peciccia, MD,** is a psychiatrist, Scientific Director at the Gaetano Benedetti Institute of Psychoanalytic Existential Psychotherapy (Assisi, Italy), member of IAGP, and President of ISPS Italy. Together with Gaetano Benedetti, he has developed the method of progressive mirror drawing. He teaches this in Italy, at the University of Perugia, in Switzerland and in Germany. He is the author of many publications concerning psychoanalytic-oriented psychotherapy of psychosis.

**Nada Perovšek Šolinc, MD,** is a psychiatrist and group analyst. She was Head of the Department for Psychiatry at the University psychiatric clinic in Ljubljana, and she has worked in the centre for psychiatric outpatients in Ljubljana. She teaches in postgraduate courses of psychotherapy, group analysis and ISPS Slovenia. Her papers are published internationally.

**Sonja Petković, MD,** is a forensic psychiatrist with education in psychotherapy. She is Head of the forensic unit in a neuropsychiatric hospital in Popovača, Croatia. Professional interests include individual and group psychotherapy of different psychotic patients with criminal backgrounds. She is co-author of several professional papers.

**Branka Restek-Petrović, MD, Ph.D.,** is a psychiatrist and group analyst. She is Head of a psychotherapeutic unit in a day hospital and co-Director in the psychiatric hospital Sveti Ivan in Zagreb, Croatia. Her professional interests include inpatient and outpatient group psychotherapy of psychotic and borderline patients, as well as early intervention in psychosis. As a senior psychotherapist and training group analyst, she organises the psychodynamic group for psychotherapy education of nursing staff, and also functions as a supervisor in group psychotherapy. She is the author of several professional papers and book chapters.

**Olga Runciman** is a psychologist and owner of the company Psycovery. She has specialised in working with people in severe distress. Psycovery is the first and only private practice in Denmark that offers therapy to people typically labeled with psychosis. She also works part-time in the innovation and developmental team in a long-term psychiatric institute. She is a registered psychiatric nurse and has worked as such for many years in psychiatry before becoming a psychologist. Learning about psychiatry from the inside out enables her to bridge the two worlds found within psychiatry; that of the psychiatric patient and that of the professionals working in psychiatry. She is greatly inspired by the many ways of communicating and is currently in the process of taking the 3-year Finnish Open Dialogue education to become a family therapist. She is a board member of: the Danish Hearing Voices Network, the Danish Psychosocial Rehabilitation network, Mad in America, International Institute for Psychiatric Drug Withdrawal, Intervoice, the International Hearing Voices Network, and Death in Psychiatry.

**Sladana Štrkalj Ivezić, MD, Ph.D.,** is a psychiatrist, subspecialist in social psychiatry and psychotherapy, group analyst, and psychodynamically oriented family, marital and partnership psychotherapist. She is Head of the Social

Psychiatry Department in the psychiatric hospital Vrapče in Zagreb, Croatia; President of the Croatian Society for Clinical Psychiatry and Psychosocial Treatment of Psychoses; Croatian representative for the European Union of Medical Specialists Board of Psychiatry; and President of the association for promotion of mental health users' organisation Svitanje. She is also co-organiser and Scientific co-Director of the School of Psychotherapy of Psychoses at the Inter-University Center, Dubrovnik. She is the author of several books, including: *Psychoeducation Between the Information and Psychotherapy*; and *Recovery from Schizophrenia and Bipolar Disorder: Rehabilitation in psychiatry – psychobiosocial model*; as well as many papers published internationally. Her interests encompass scientific projects and research in the different fields of genetic, psychopharmacotherapeutic, stigma, psychotherapy and social psychiatry.

**Thomas Styron** is a clinical psychologist and Associate Professor of Psychiatry at the Yale School of Medicine. He serves as Executive Director of the Community Services Network of Greater New Haven, a collaborative of 18 community-based not-for-profit organisations which provide a broad array of integrated community supports for individuals with serious mental illness, such as housing, employment and social opportunities. His research and teaching focus on best practices in the area of recovery-oriented care for individuals with serious mental illnesses. Based at the Connecticut Mental Health Center, a public psychiatric hospital under the auspices of Yale's Department of Psychiatry, and the Connecticut Department of Mental Health and Addiction Services, he also oversees the psychology training programme for the center's outpatient services division.

**Dani Tost, MS, Ph.D.,** is Professor at Universitat Politècnica de Catalunya, Barcelona, and also Director of the Research Center of Bioengineering. Her research focuses on medical applications of computer graphics, specifically serious games and gamifications for training, diagnosis, rehabilitation and assessment. She has been leader of various national and European research projects, and has published internationally.

**Lina Tost, MB, Ph.D.,** graduated in medicine and surgery (Barcelona University, 1983), and then specialised in psychiatry and psychosomatics. She has worked in the Psychiatric Hospital of Tenerife and, as a liaison psychiatrist, in Hospital De La Candelaria in Tenerife. As Head of a mental health centre, she organises different therapies for patients with schizophrenia. She has published several papers on psychiatry. Recently, she has co-authored an evaluation report on health technologies of the Spanish National Health System on group psychotherapy for persons with schizophrenia.

**Ivan Urlić, MD, Ph.D.,** is a neuropsychiatrist, psychoanalytic psychotherapist and group analyst. He is Professor of Psychiatry and Psychological Medicine at the Medical School, University of Split, Croatia. He is founder member of

IGA Zagreb (Croatia) and IGA Bologna (Italy), where he is training analyst and supervisor. In 2004 he was Foulkes Lecturer. He was Chairperson of the European Group Analytic Training Institutions Network (EGATIN), board member of GASi, IAGP and ISPS International, and organised the 17th ISPS International Congress on psychological approaches to psychoses, Dubrovnik, Croatia, 2011. As ISPS Croatia co-founder, he is also its Vice President and co-organises the School of Psychotherapy of Psychoses, held yearly in Dubrovnik. He is founder of the Regional Center for Psycho-trauma in Split, and organised the first WHO training in PTSD in Croatia. He is the author of many papers, and lectures in Croatian and internationally in English, Italian and French.

**Truus van den Brink** is a community psychiatrist, co-worker of Margreet de Pater who developed the Transmural Family Guidance in Altrecht. Together they presented several workshops at national and international congresses concerning family work and how to train mental health workers in the Netherlands to work with patients and their families.

**Editha Vučić, MD,** is a psychiatrist, whose professional interest covers inpatient and outpatient group psychotherapy of patients with psychosis and other severely disturbed patients, and in forensic patients.

**Richard Youins** is a person who is 5½ years drug-free and in recovery from bipolar disorder. With the support and love of his family and work colleagues, he has been able to pursue all eight dimensions of wellness. He co-leads a home group while continuing to work on himself and finding ways to make what seemed to be impossibilities possible, including giving back to those who helped him and taking the kindness and generosity of a warm and supportive community.

**Tija Žarković Palijan, MD,** is a psychiatrist in the psychiatric hospital Dr. Ivan Barbot in Popovača, Croatia, where she has been Head of the Alcoholics Department since 1985, Head of the Forensic Psychiatry Department since 1994, and Coordinator of the Institute for Forensic Psychiatry. Her doctoral thesis was entitled 'Personality traits of alcoholic offenders and non-offenders of crimes', and she has also co-authored *Forensic Psychiatry* volumes 1, 2 and 3 (2007, 2009 and 2011). As well as participating in congresses presenting general, special and forensic psychiatry in Croatia and abroad, she holds certificates in psychotherapy and various other alternative psychiatric methods of treatment.

# Foreword by Brian Martindale

'Let's Get Together'

(Chet Powers, 1960s)

Have I gone mad? I'm afraid so, but let me tell you something, the best people usually are.

(*Alice in Wonderland*, directed by Tim Burton, 2010)

A crucial ingredient of a therapeutic group is the finding of hope; especially hope that one can be accepted by fellow human beings. This book, which focusses on groups for those who have experienced psychosis, will inspire hope in any open-minded reader, whatever his or her knowledge or experience of therapeutic groups. Those somewhat disillusioned with contemporary mental health services will find a wonderful smorgasbord of applications for group therapies in many different situations with patient or client groups who are vulnerable to 'psychotic' experiences. Readers working *within* contemporary services will be stimulated by the range of possibilities for developing group therapies in these contexts. Those who feel that the obstacles and resistances of their statutory mental health systems are too great will also be inspired by accounts of groups working outside of those systems, such as those within the Hearing Voices Movement and specific peer-centered group projects.

I was impressed that the editors chose to 'converse' right at the beginning with those who might see themselves as a 'doubting Thomas' about group therapies. This reflects the overall respectful tone of the book, which is not to portray group therapies as a kind of panacea for all, but as a certain way to organise a variety of group settings so that they can improve the chances for a good number of people (who experience psychosis) to have a more meaningful life, especially in the attachments and involvements they may be able to create with fellow human beings. Yet the book does not ignore why groups may be less successful or even toxic for some. It addresses how these possibilities can be either anticipated in careful group selection, or attended to within a group when negativity threatens to surface in a way that could be destructive to the group or to individual members.

By examining the historical evolution of group therapies for those experiencing psychosis, the reader will gain an excellent contemporary perspective (maybe even on their own mental health service). Digesting this background will support the realisation of the importance of group therapies being carried out within a supportive organisational context, and the relational work needed to achieve such an environment. There is no place for messianic leaders or messianic approaches to group work in this book!

This book is also commendable for its welcoming of group approaches from a number of theoretical perspectives; yet rarely does theory dominate. That is not to say that the reader will not come away without having internalised many of the common factors that are specific to successful *group* therapies of all persuasions. Paradoxically, these are often called (in an unfortunately debasing way) non-specific factors, and they include such vital factors as universality, the instillation of hope, and altruism. These factors need to be distinguished from the additional specific factors of a particular group approach, such as a focus on voices, using the media of the arts therapies, or relational insight-orientated group therapy.

In any therapy, the question of a person revealing their crucial personal issues is both central and complex. Where psychosis and a group context are concerned, the factors might seem exponentially more complex and daunting and so most people, if asked, would prefer individual therapy. This book puts these anxieties into perspective, when it discusses the subjective reality that is felt to be objective by the person, and its unfolding in the context of multiple subjectivities and multiple objectivities of the group. This underscores the necessity of the group facilitator(s) to be fully grounded in group understandings and skills in order to prevent carrying out individual work in a group context.

The authors, from a number of different countries, have clearly been successful in delivering groups in their settings – readers may have to contain their envy if their setting is sorely limited in the provision of group therapies. However, we must hope that in the decades to come there will be an increasing availability of group therapies; a setting so relevant to the difficulties of people in living a socially integrated life. The past dominance of the neurobiological explanation is beginning to wane, and the reintegration of psychosocial factors and personal histories offers hope that the world is indeed becoming more 'rounded'.

I want to end with a quote from the book that led me to select the lyrics of Chet Powers and the words from *Alice in Wonderland* at the beginning of my foreword:

> Nothing has proven to be as potent a response to stigma and discrimination as being introduced to a living, breathing example of a person who has shattered the negative stereotypes associated with having a mental illness or an addiction. By their very presence in the group, peer leaders already challenge members to imagine and come to believe in the possibility of having better or fuller lives.

The editors are to be congratulated on bringing together such a talented group of authors from the western hemisphere. I hope the book will become mandatory reading and discussion for all who train within the mental health field. It should also be of interest to those with responsibility for the development of mental health services and to those who provide alternative services in the community.

*Brian Martindale*
*Former President of ISPS*

# Foreword by Brian Koehler

If you want to go fast, go alone. If you want to go far, go together.
(African Proverb)

Human beings have survived and thrived through the centuries by joining together in groups to accomplish necessary and/or rewarding tasks for living. As pointed out by Cacioppo and Patrick (2008), feeling isolated can undermine our ability to trust others and to think clearly: indeed, evolution has formed us to feel good and secure when connected to others. To be excluded from the group or community can be very harmful to people, e.g., the phenomena of somatic or psychic death through social exclusion/isolation. Loneliness has a psychobiological and immunological cost. Social relationships, potentially imbued with significant anxiety and fear of abandonment, can be growth promoting, reparative and even life saving.

In this book, Ivan Urlić and Manuel González de Chávez initiate the reader into some of the reasons for the group therapeutic efficacy for persons experiencing states of psychosis (see page xxvi):

*universality* (discovering you are not the only one person with the problem), *hope* (seeing that change and improvement is possible in other members) and *acceptance* by others (despite the problem).

Universality could help to decrease the sense of shame, social isolation and exclusion, as well as the stigmatisation these persons can experience. A neurology applies to hope and hopelessness, as a robust research literature demonstrates. Hope has been shown to be necessary for recovery. Acceptance by other persons also helps to counteract the loneliness, isolation and low self-esteem these individuals may have experienced in their lives. Urlić and González de Chávez also introduce, in the Preface, the potential negative effects of introducing a person into group therapy who has a deep mistrust of other people, is feeling overwhelmed, and is struggling with defences against psychotic anxieties (Bion, 1961).

The organisation of this much-needed and scholarly volume consists of two parts. The first is comprised of an overview of the history, research, therapeutic factors, and the factors involved in the creation of therapy groups for persons struggling with psychotic states and experiences. The second part is comprised of a vast array of clinically relevant approaches to group therapy with persons with the lived experience of psychosis. These include: psychoanalytic and psycho-dynamic, psychoeducation, groups in therapeutic communities, groups in early intervention services, CBT, multi-family groups, peer-led groups, groups based on the Hearing Voices Movement, and groups using creative arts therapies.

Almost 20 years ago, I worked as a group therapist for persons with the lived experience of psychosis for many years. On a daily basis, I led or co-led group therapies in inpatient and outpatient settings, including long-term daily groups within a state psychiatric hospital. One of the principles of therapeutic communities – 'patients helping patients' – was very evident and also inspiring. The degree to which group members were very perceptive and helpful towards their peers was impressive to say the least. It reminds me of observations made by Pfaff (2015), that from a neurobiological perspective we are biased towards behaving altruistically towards others. During these years, I observed the validity of what the editors and authors of this volume have proposed as the multiple factors underlying therapeutic action: altruism, universality, cohesion, acceptance, passive vicarious and active interpersonal learning, understanding and insight, psychoeducation, catharsis, mobilisation of hope, self-disclosure and reality testing, among others.

I was definitely changed as a result of these intensive group therapy experiences, in conjunction with my work as an individual psychotherapist within these settings, along the lines articulated by the great interpersonal psychiatrist Harry Stack Sullivan (2013, p. 18) who commented:

> In most general terms, we are all *much more simply human than otherwise*, be we happy and successful, contented and detached, miserable and mentally disordered, or whatever.

Each group was unique in their membership, but similar themes would emerge: concerns with self-esteem, relationships, existential issues, trauma, autonomy and control issues. I read a great deal of the literature on group psychotherapy and milieu therapy with persons with the lived experience of psychosis because at that time people in a state psychiatric hospital would stay for longer periods of time, for better or worse. This volume fills a need for those of us who value the range and depth of group psychotherapies for persons experiencing psychotic states.

I, as well as many authors represented in this volume, found the work of Irving Yalom particularly helpful for inpatient and outpatient group therapy. In his recent autobiography, Yalom (2017, p. 202) noted:

> I began by visiting group meetings on inpatient wards at leading psychiatric hospitals around the country. I found confusion everywhere: not even the best-known academic hospitals had an effective inpatient group program [. . .] No one seemed to be getting much benefit from these groups, and

attrition was high. An entirely different strategy was needed [. . .] I entirely gave up on the idea of continuity from one meeting to the next and developed a new paradigm: the life of the group would be a single session [. . .]

Yalom developed an approach to inpatient and outpatient group psychotherapy that asked each person to work on an interpersonal issue in a group. After the group meeting ended, a group of observers who had used a one-way mirror, entered the room and, for 10 minutes, openly discussed the meeting while the 'patients' observed from an outer circle. In the last 10 minutes of the group, the group members responded to the observers' post-group discussion. Yalom believed that the results of this approach were better than when members focused on why they were hospitalised. Interestingly, Yalom reported a survey in which the 'patients' rated the last 20 minutes as the most worthwhile of the group experience. This seems to me to be somewhat analogous to some processes that occur in Open Dialogue in which people in the social network, as well as 'therapists', openly speak their thoughts to each other.

This volume is a Babette's Feast for those who wish to savour the depth and breadth of approaches to group psychotherapy with persons experiencing distressing psychotic states.

*Brian Koehler*
*New York University and Teachers College, Columbia University*

## References

Bion, W.R. (1961) *Experiences in Groups.* London: Tavistock Publications.

Cacioppo, J.T. and Patrick, W. (2008) *Loneliness: Human nature and the need for social connection.* New York: Norton & Company.

Pfaff, D.W. (2015) *The Altruistic Brain: How we are naturally good.* Oxford: Oxford University Press.

Sullivan, H.S. (2013) *The Interpersonal Theory of Psychiatry.* London: Tavistock Publications.

Yalom, I.D. (2017) *Becoming Myself: A psychiatrist's memoir.* New York: Basic Books.

# Preface

This book is intended for anyone interested in how groups can help someone suffering from the distressing or disabling effects of psychosis. This includes those already engaged in this work (group analysts, CBT practitioners, family therapists, etc.), those interested in using groups but not yet doing so, those who are participating as a member of a group or thinking about doing this, and concerned family members and friends of someone with psychosis. Our aim therefore has been to produce a book of interest to, and accessible to, all these readers. Inevitably we will fall short of this ideal, but we have tried to approach it by encompassing as wide a range of group approaches to psychosis as we can within a single book, and by asking our contributors to use language which as far as possible is non-technical and does not assume prior knowledge of their particular theory or therapeutic methods.

However, the reader will notice that a number of chapters are written from a psychodynamic or group-analytic point of view. This is for two reasons. Firstly, this is the shared background of the co-editors, so we naturally have an interest in presenting these approaches. Secondly, from a historical perspective, psychoanalytic interest in the treatment of psychosis predated other therapeutic approaches by several decades in the twentieth century (as witnessed in the origins of ISPS), and in many countries a psychodynamic approach to psychosis still predominates over other more recent psychological approaches. By inviting contributions from a range of countries where therapeutic groups are offered to people experiencing psychosis, we are reflecting the current range of practice in those countries.

To those with limited experience of therapeutic groups, or none at all, certain questions may arise that precede any concerns about the relative merits of different approaches. Questions like: Won't being in a group with other people with problems make an individual worse? Won't someone with paranoia feel more threatened by being in a group? Won't someone with a shaky grasp of reality become more disturbed in a group that delves into his or her unconscious motives? We will attempt to give a brief answer here to each of these very common concerns, although fuller discussion may be found in the chapters that follow.

Does being in a group with other people with similar problems make an individual's own problems worse? The short answer is no. There is plenty of evidence that group therapy is effective (Blackmore, et al., 2012). A more nuanced answer is that important therapeutic factors in groups include *universality* (discovering you are not the only one with the problem), *hope* (seeing that change and improvement is possible in other members) and *acceptance* by others (despite the problem). Of course, being in a group can also be a negative experience. People can feel bullied or rejected by groups. The therapeutic factors need to be brought into play, and negative factors nipped in the bud, by a skilful and sensitive group therapist or facilitator. This book is an overview of many models of group work, not a training manual, and anyone proposing to use groups in their therapeutic work is strongly advised to ensure they are well trained and supervised within the model of their choice.

Won't someone with paranoia feel more threatened by being in a group? The answer is probably yes, and strong paranoid ideas would be a contra-indication for group therapy. Group therapy is not a panacea, and while there are positive reasons for offering it, such as the therapeutic factors mentioned above, there are also reasons to not offer it, where negative reactions are likely to prevent the potential benefits.

Won't someone with a shaky grasp of reality become more disturbed in a group that delves into members' unconscious motives? The answer here is more complex. As a rule of thumb one should say that it depends on the phase of the member's psychosis (Fuller, 2013). The therapist or facilitator should avoid exploring a member's underlying fears or wishes during the early or crisis phase, when the individual is preoccupied with survival in the face of overwhelming experiences. When the individual is more settled, exploration of the underlying meaning of their experiences may be of considerable value in helping to reduce the risk of further psychotic episodes, and the value of the group arises in the opportunity it provides for members to learn from each other, support one another and contribute to each other's learning. Beyond this rule of thumb there are techniques, such as Open Dialogue, not presented in this book, that explore underlying family conflicts at the earliest possible opportunity before positions have become fixed. Perhaps the simplest guideline is that, whatever group techniques are used, the therapist's task is to maintain members' anxieties at a tolerable level.

The book is divided into two parts. The first part comprises four chapters that explore general aspects of group work with psychosis, covering its history, evaluation, research methodologies, group therapeutic factors and how groups are created and set up. The second part comprises sixteen chapters that introduce the reader to a wide range of different types of groups. The expanding range of group work with psychosis is reflected in the diversity of approaches in this section. As mentioned above there is a strong presence of psychodynamic and group-analytic approaches, reflecting their importance in the development of group therapies for psychosis and also in the mental health services in several member countries of ISPS. There are chapters on psychoeducation groups, groups in an early intervention service, cognitive behavioural groups, multi-family groups, peer support and hearing voices groups, and groups in the arts therapies. The settings for these groups include the community, outpatient clinic hospital wards and a forensic service.

We believe that the range of methods, models and settings presented in this book points to the vigour and creativity of this growing field, and we hope readers will find much to interest, inform and even inspire them.

*Ivan Urlić and Manuel González de Chávez*

## References

Blackmore, C., Tantum, D., Parry, G. and Chambers, E. (2012) Report on a systematic review of the efficacy and clinical effectiveness of group analysis and analytic/dynamic group psychotherapy. *Group Analysis,* 45(1), 46–69.

Fuller, P.R. (2013) *Surviving, Existing, or Living.* London: Routledge.

# Acknowledgements

We as authors and editors are grateful to Dr Brian Martindale, the former President of ISPS, who, during the 17th International Congress for the Psychological Treatments of the Schizophrenias and other Psychoses in Dubrovnik, Croatia, 2011, initiated the idea of a book on the use of groups in treating persons suffering from psychoses.

We are very grateful to all our patients in group psychotherapy who made it possible to better understand their psychotic experiences and the ways we could help them in their crises.

We would like to express our recognition to all our colleagues and members of the therapeutic teams, for their compassion, patience and dedication in approaching and working with patients suffering from psychotic disorders, and to their family members. In return they entrusted us with their full confidence, respect and their deepest feelings and specific perceptions.

Our acknowledgement goes to the contributors of this book. They were chosen as prominent professionals, who contribute their expertise and publications in order to further the knowledge and practice of using group settings in the frame of the comprehensive treatment of people suffering from psychoses.

We greatly appreciate the cooperability and affability of the publisher and its team for their highly professional performance in organising the process of publication of this book. Our thanks also to Mrs Antoslava Vukas, who was committed to the technical work on this book for years.

Last but not least, we are especially thankful to our families for their patience and support throughout the years of our professional work and during the creation of this book.

*Ivan Urlić and Manuel González de Chávez*

Part I

# Overview of group psychotherapies for people suffering from psychoses

Chapter 1

# History of group psychotherapy for patients with psychoses

*Manuel González de Chávez*

Groups are potentially dangerous places and therefore unsuitable for therapeutic purposes.

(letter from Freud to Trigant Burrow: Pertegato and Pertegato, 2013: p. xxxiii)

First you will get the sociologists, then the social psychologists, then the general practitioners, then the plain people, but you will never live to see the day when psychiatrists will accept group psychotherapy.

(William Alanson White to Jacob L. Moreno: Moreno, 1989)

The beginnings of group psychotherapy were not exempt from encountering many resistances, as shown by the attitude of Freud and the observation of William Alanson White on the psychiatrists of their times. With the exception of some group and theater–therapeutic experiences in the nineteenth century in some psychiatric asylums, such as those of Glasgow (Hunter and Macalpine, 1963), Kiev or St Petersburg (Blatner, 2000), it was during the first decades of the twentieth century when social interest regarding knowledge of groups, their dynamics and possible functionality, began to develop (Strodtbeck and Hare, 1954).

The history of group psychotherapy in the psychoses is therefore connected to that of sociological and psychosocial research of the groups in addition to that of the history of group therapy in general and to the more extensive history of the psychotherapy of the psychoses. Three stages in the history of group psychotherapy in the psychoses can be differentiated: (1) a first stage of *initiation* of these therapies, which would correspond to the first half of the twentieth century; (2) a second stage of *expansion* of the group therapies in psychoses, which took place from the 1950s to the 1990s; and (3) a third stage of *consolidation* of these therapies during the last 30 years.

## Initiation

In the first decades of the twentieth century, the groups that were started in the hospital setting with psychotic patients were either didactic, with lectures, illustrative cases and other pedagogical procedures, or recreational and ludic, with social activities to promote interaction of the patients. The first publication on group therapy of dementia precox was by Edward W. Lazell (1921), who described the experience that occurred in one of the most advanced American hospitals of the time, Saint Elizabeth's Hospital of Washington, directed by William Allanson White. In that hospital, individual psychotherapy of the psychoses had already begun with Edward J. Kempf, a pioneer and precursor of Harry S. Sullivan, who worked in the same centre years later. Lazell had already carried out individual didactic therapeutic interventions in the style of Kempf and made the proposal to W.A. White of organising some wards with selected patients to add the 'group method' to therapeutic activities, obtaining 'rewarding results'. The groups included conferences, lectures or cases, followed by group discussion. In those times, homosexuality was in the origin of dementia precox: an aggressive homosexuality derived from the hebephrenics, and a sumissive one from the paranoids. The group method made it possible for the patients to speak about their lives and to channel their sexuality towards heterosexual objectives. Lazell was an enthusiastic sponsor during the entire first half of the twentieth century of didactic group psychotherapies tackling important problems and difficulties (Lazell, 1945).

Later, in the third decade of the twentieth century, group therapies with psycho-analytic approaches and concepts began in the US (Kaplan and Sadock, 1972), although Alfred Adler had initiated group experiences years earlier in Europe. At this time, group therapies with psychotic patients were conducted in the most advanced American centres (Abrahan and Varon, 1953; Frank, 1952; Standish, et al., 1952).

The pioneers of group therapies with schizophrenic patients faced all the uncertainties and lack of knowledge regarding these disorders, together with those of the new context of the group therapies. Many were enthusiastic young people without experience or bibliographic references, who did not fully know how to act with these patients gathered into a group. They wondered about the objectives and priorities of group therapy. Socialisation of the patients? Lifting them out of isolation? Helping them to verbalise their experiences? Regarding the size of the groups: the entire ward, or small, homogeneous, mixed, acute or chronic groups? They discussed how the institution affected the groups and the groups the insti-tution. Obviously, they also questioned their own role as therapists: teaching, mobilising or listening? Passive or directive? Allowing the patients to speak freely? Giving priority to each patient or to the global functioning of the group? They were interested in achieving an environment where the patients listened to each other. Was it necessary to speak in the group only about the 'healthy aspects' of each individual or also to include the psychotic experiences? Only about the 'here and now' or also about the 'there and then'? They were concerned about how to handle aggressivity or passivity of the patients, hyperactivity and verboseness of some of them, and silences and autism of others. How to cope with fear, distrust, hopelessness and suicidal ideas in the group? What to do with the verbalisation of the psychotic experiences – minimise them, ignore them, listen to them, interpret them, or try to understand them?

Around the mid-twentieth century, many group initiatives with psychotic patients had been performed: didactic and psychoeducation groups, psychodramas, groups with puppet theaters, music therapy, dance therapy, groups with recreational and rehabilitation activities, psychoanalytic, interpersonal or psychosocial groups, hospital and outpatient groups, for acute or chronic patients, family groups, and homogeneous or mixed groups with neurotic patients. The first observations of group dynamics and processes had already been made with these patients, as well as short-term results and evaluations, and some of the combined therapies and comparative studies of group and individual therapies, or patients treated with or without group therapy (see Meiers, 1945; Stotsky and Zolik, 1965).

The study of the groups, from sociology or social psychology perspectives, also advanced from decision making or interpersonal influence to becoming interested in other subjects, such as structure and group environment (Lewin, 1947). Nonetheless, it is an extra issue of *Sociometry* (entitled 'Group psychotherapy: A symposium', 1945), the journal founded by J.L. Moreno, which offers us the best view of the state of the group therapies as a whole in the mid-twentieth century. This issue also includes a series of articles from American and English military psychiatrists and presents some of the keys to the subsequent expansion of group dynamics, when they were accepted and incorporated with enthusiasm by these democratic armed forces. It was the military psychiatry of these countries, before, during and after the Second World War, that gave a decisive impulse to the group practices and therapies. In England, for example, the subsequent development of the therapeutic communities, social psychiatry or group analysis could not be understood without the military hospital of Northfield, where Rickman, Foulkes, Bion, Maxwell Jones, Joshua Bierer and many others coincided in group practice (Harrison, 2000).

## Expansion

Publications on group therapy in general and applied to psychotic patients specifically, multiplied exponentially beginning with the Second World War (Corsini and Putzey, 1957), and continued to do so in subsequent decades. At the end of the 1980s, there were more than five thousand articles on group psychotherapy in the psychoses published in the English language alone (Lubin and Lubin, 1987) and it must be supposed that more existed in other languages. Two journals dedicated to group therapies – *International Journal of Group Psychotherapy* and *Group Analysis* – stand out for having collected articles dedicated to group psychotherapy in the psychoses.

The second half of the twentieth century was enormously productive for group therapies in general and also for those specifically dedicated to psychotic patients. The therapeutic contexts became diversified beyond the hospital setting, with the new care organisation advocated by community psychiatry. Groups were dedicated to rehabilitation, in its diverse aspects, performed in centres and day hospitals or in therapeutic communities, and the outpatient groups in mental health centres, which now assumed a new decisive role in care.

Many group therapy practices with psychotic patients were broadly developed: psychoeducation, psychodynamic, interpersonal, supportive, insight, social skills and problem solving, and other diverse models to which cognitive behavioural group therapies were incorporated in subsequent years. The first group psychotherapy manuals – by Klapman (1946), Corsini (1957) and Johnson (1963) – were published, and some had chapters dedicated to psychoses (Johnson, 1963), which would later become more common in major group psychotherapy manuals such as Kaplan and Sadock (1971). The first books on group psychotherapy for inpatients (Yalom, 1983; Rice and Rutan, 1987) and in children with psychotic problems (Speers and Lansing, 1965) were also published. Family therapies, which were expanded in these decades, also had their group equivalent with multi-family therapies. In addition, research in group therapies for patients with diverse diagnoses and also in schizophrenia proliferated, evaluating results for inpatients or outpatients, and comparing them with other therapeutic alternatives or in therapies combined with other psychosocial interventions (Parloff and Dies, 1977; González de Chávez, 2009).

All the individual, family group and institutional therapies with psychotic patients expanded in the second half of the twentieth century, and with them the interest for training of professionals and the indications of said therapies, in addition to their interactions, comparative studies, therapeutic procedures and the development of care programmes (see Alanen, Silver and González de Chávez, 2006).

## Consolidation

The third and last stage of the history of group therapies in the psychoses began in the last decades of the last century and has continued up to the present. It began with the publication of the first books entirely dedicated to group psychotherapy in psychotic patients (Ascher-Svanun and Krause, 1991; Kanas, 1996; Schermer and Pines, 1999; Stone, 1996). This is a stage of maturity, consolidation, adaptation, integration and re-evaluation of these therapies. The need to integrate perspectives and models is suggested at this time, as simultaneously occurs in psychotherapies in general. Processes of adaptation take place: of adapting to the organisation of the public services and to the funding forms of the care; to new therapeutic contexts with psychotic patients, such as therapeutic communities; and to new strategies such as early intervention, and the concepts of empowerment and recovery for persons who have gone through psychotic experiences that make group dynamics the guiding force that carries them to their objectives. These final group experiences (self-help group, peer-support group, recovery group, etc.) are enriching group therapies with psychotic patients, especially those of persons who hear voices, and these networks are already extended in all the countries of the world.

The current stage of development of group therapies in general and in group therapy of psychoses specifically is also characterised by a special emphasis on: the evaluation of these therapies; the choice of the quality indicators; the methodology of the publications or trials, their statistical processing, sample sizes and control groups; and on all the investigation that refers to their efficacy, indications, processes or mechanisms of change and specific therapeutic factors. They are keys in the future development, implementation and differentiation of these therapies (Furhiman and Burlingame, 1994; Burlingame, Kircher and Taylor, 1994; Manor, 2009; Tost, Hernandez and González de Chávez, 2012).

## What have we learned in one century of group psychotherapy of the psychoses?

The group psychotherapy of the psychoses has a century of history. It is practised worldwide, in institutions and organisations of all types, in many care programmes, with many modalities and approaches, and in a very heterogeneous wide range of persons with psychotic experiences, biographic evolutions and distinct characteristics. There are already tens of thousands of articles in scientific journals, and monographic books on this therapeutic practice continue to be published periodically (Radcliffe, et al., 2010; Lecomte, Leclerc and Wilkes, 2016). However, we must not get lost in the boundless forest of many local circumstances and characteristics of organisations, settings, formats, techniques, therapeutic training or styles. Rather, we should remember what this century of history of group psychotherapy in the psychoses has taught us. We could sum it up as follows:

- It is useful to perform group psychotherapies on patients with psychotic experiences working as a team, within an institutional context, in accordance with the usual demands of the centre, and forming a part of a more global care programme.
- We must never forget that the greatest part of the life of the patient occurs outside of the group, with other interactions, relationships, objective and concerns.
- The group, in order to be therapeutic, must be held in a safe place for the patient, and not one that is a source of problems and conflicts.
- The therapeutic process takes its time and has stages: for example, contact, self-disclosure, understanding, integration and change.
- As therapists, we must work with an open mind regarding the group reality, and without previous and closed hypotheses on the psychotic experiences of its members.
- The different approaches or group techniques should be adapted to the needs of the patients because they are less relevant than the common group therapeutic factors.
- The help provided by the group psychotherapy is not directly addressed to the suppression of the psychotic experiences, but rather to the dynamics, relational

patterns, conflicts, coping strategies or defense mechanisms that trigger and make them possible.

- For the help to be most effective in group psychotherapy in the psychoses, it should be initiated as early as possible. In this way, the patient can become desingularised from the first episode, quickly calling into question the subjective character of one's psychotic experiences, accepting his/her disorders and problems, abandoning the defensive autism, and establishing therapeutic relationships more quickly.
- The therapy group is often the psychotic patient's only reference group, which can facilitate a more objective view of oneself, contrasting and questioning the psychotic identities and blocking the development of delusion convictions or beliefs in the truthfulness of the psychotic experiences lived.
- The therapy group is a socialising, motivating and altruistic support for the patient that permits him/her to better know his/her recovery progress, helping the patient to fight against depression, demoralisation and stigma, and aiding the patient to be able to approach, analyse and improve his/her problems in interpersonal and familial relationships.

Knowing, stressing, demonstrating and disseminating the therapeutic importance of the group dynamics among the mental health professionals and in the population in general, and to immerse in the cultural values of the dominant individualism, is an immediate objective in order to ensure access of the psychotic patients to group therapeutic contexts. Such access permits them to break away from their isolation, and to communicate, share and try to understand their experiences, to evaluate them, face or overcome them with dignity, and to achieve or continue with a possible and realistic life project.

## References

Abrahan, J. and Varon, E. (1953) *Maternal Dependency and Schizophrenia.* New York: International University Press.

Alanen, Y.O., Silver, A.L. and González de Chávez, M. (2006) *Fifty Years of Humanistic Treatment of Psychoses*. Madrid: ISPS & Fundación para la investigación y Tratamiento de la Esquizofrenia y otras Psicosis.

Ascher-Svanun, H. and Krause, A. (1991) *Psychoeducational Groups for Patients with Schizophrenia*. Maryland: Aspen Publication.

Blatner, A. (2000) *Foundations of Psychodrama: History, theory and practice.* New York: Springer.

Burlingame, G.M., Kircher, J.C. and Taylor, S. (1994) 'Methodological considerations in group psychotherapy research: Past, present and future practices' (pp. 41–80) in A. Fuhriman and G.M. Burlingame (Eds), *Handbook of Group Psychotherapy.* New York: Wiley.

Corsini, R.J. (1957) *Methods of Group Pyschotherapy.* New York: McGraw-Hill.

Corsini, R.J. and Putzey, L.J. (1957) Bibliography of group psychotherapy 1906–1956. *Psychodrama and Group Psychotherapy Monographs, 29.*

Frank, J. (1952) 'Group psychotherapy with chronic hospitalized schizophrenic' in E.B. Brody and F.C. Redlich (Eds), *Psychotherapy with Schizophrenics*. New York: International University Press.

Furhiman, A. and Burlingame, G.M. (1994) 'Group psychotherapy: Research and practice' (pp. 3–40) in *Handbook of Group Psychotherapy*. New York: Wiley.

González de Chávez, M. (2009) 'Group psychotherapy and schizophrenia' in Y.O. Alanen, M. González de Chávez, A.L. Silver and B. Martindale (Eds), *Psychotherapeutic Approaches to Schizophrenic Psychosis: Past, present and future*. London: Routledge.

Harrison, T. (2000) *Bion, Rickman, Foulkes and the Northfield Experiments: Advancing on a differenet front*. London: Jessica Kingsley.

Hunter, R. and Macalpine, I. (1963) 'Glasgow asylum for lunatics. Fifth annual report of directors 1819. Patients in groups' (pp. 746–747) in *Three Hundred Years of Psychiatry 1535–1860*. New York: Oxford University Press.

Johnson, J.A. (1963) *Group Therapy: A practical approach*. New York: McGraw-Hill.

Kanas, N. (1996) *Group Therapy for Schizophrenic Patients*. Washington: American Psychiatric Press.

Kaplan, H.I. and Sadock, B.J. (1971) *Comprehensive Group Psychotherapy*, 1st edition. Baltimore: Williams and Wilkins.

Kaplan, H.I. and Sadock, B.J. (1972) *The Origins of Group Psychoanalysis*. New York: Jason Aronson.

Klapman, J.W. (1946) *Group Psychotherapy: Theory and practice*. Washington: Heinemann Medical Books.

Lazell, E.W. (1921) The group treatment of dementia precox. *Psychoanalytic Review*, 8, 168–179.

Lazell, E.W. (1945) Group psychotherapy. *Sociometry*, 8(3/4), 101–107.

Lecomte, T., Leclerc, C. and Wilkes, T. (2016) *Group CBT for Psychosis*. Oxford: Oxford University Press.

Lewin, K. (1947) Frontiers in group dynamics: Concept, method and reality in social science. Equilibrium and social change. *Human Relations*, 1, 5–41.

Lubin, B. and Lubin, A.W. (1987) 'Comprehensive index of group psychotherapy writings' in *Monograph 2. American Group Psychotherapy Association*. New York: International University Press.

Manor, O. (2009) *Groupwork Research*. London: Whiting & Birch Ltd.

Meiers, J.I. (1945) Origin and development of group psychotherapy. *Sociometry*, 8(3/4), 261–296.

Moreno, J.L. (1945) Group psychotherapy: A symposium. *Sociometry*, 8(3/4).

Moreno, J.L. (1989) The autobiography of J.L. Moreno M.D. *Journal of Group Psychotherapy, Psychodrama and Sociometry, 42(1), 96.*

Parloff, M. and Dies, R. (1977) Group psychotherapy outcome research 1966–1975. *International Journal of Group Psychotherapy*, 27, 281–319.

Pertegato, E.G. and Pertegato, G.O. (2013) *From Psychoanalysis to Group Analysis: The pioneering work of Trigant Burrow*. London: Karnac Books.

Radcliffe, J., Hajek, K., Carson, J. and Manor, O. (2010) *Psychological Groupwork with Acute Psychiatric Inpatients*. London: Whiting & Birch Ltd.

Rice, C.A. and Rutan, J.S. (1987) *Inpatient Group Psychotherapy*. New York: Macmillan.

Schermer, V.L. and Pines, M. (1999) *Group Psychotherapy of the Psychoses*. London: Jessica Kingsley.

Speers, R.W. and Lansing, C. (1965) *Group Therapy in Childhood Psychosis.* Chapel Hill: The University of North Carolina Press.

Standish, C.T., Gurri, J., Semrad, E.V. and Day, M. (1952) Some difficulties in group psychotherapy with psychotics. *American Journal of Psychiatry,* 109(4), 283–286.

Stone, W.N. (1996) *Group Psychotherapy for People with Chronic Mental Illness.* New York: Guilford Press.

Stotsky, B.A. and Zolik, E.S. (1965) Group psychotherapy with psychotics: 1921–1963 – A review. *International Journal of Group Psychotherapy,* 16, 321–344.

Strodtbeck, F.L. and Hare, P. (1954) Bibliography of small group research (From 1900 through 1953). *Sociometry,* 17(2), 107–178.

Tost, L., Hernández, C.B and González de Chávez, M. (2012) 'Psicoterapia de grupo en la esquizofrenia durante los últimos 25 años. Una revisión basada en la evidencia' ['Group psychotherapy for schizophrenia during the last 25 years: An evidence-based review'] (pp. 305–359) in M. González de Chávez (Ed), *25 Años de Psicoterapia de Grupo en las Psicosis* [*25 Years of Group Psychotherapy of Psychosis*]. Madrid: Fundación para la Investigación y Tratamiento de la Esquizofrenia y otras Psicosis.

Yalom, I. (1983) *Inpatient Group Psychotherapy.* New York: Basic Books.

# Chapter 2

# Limitations of nomothetic procedures for group psychotherapy in psychosis

## A gamified approach to Yalom's therapeutic factors Q-sort

*Lina Tost, Dani Tost, Cecilio Hernández,*
*Manuel González de Chávez*

## Introduction

Group therapy still remains one of the less advanced research topics among existing treatments for psychosis. Nevertheless, over the years, several authors have tried to identify key elements of group therapy for psychosis and have reported success with this therapeutic approach, showing favorable comparisons of group versus individual treatments. Kanas (1986) pointed out that schizophrenic group therapies are cost effective, lower the rates of re-admission to hospital and are valued by patients. Others authors, such as Chazan (2001) and Urlić (2010), report that groups ease the learning of communication, testing reality or being accepted as an equal, and it aids the feeling of being helpful to others. González de Chávez (2008) outlined that the therapeutic potential of the group for psychotic patients comes from the mirroring phenomenon and from the fact that therapeutic factors are horizontally multiplied and reciprocally boosted by group dynamics. Today, most psychiatric departments in the world assume group therapy as a complement to their general approach.

Nevertheless important limitations on providing evidences about its benefits still exist. The suitability of nomothetic methods to assess psychosocial interventions, where the subjective components are enormously significant and are often overlooked by quantitative methods used in evidence-based medicine (EBM), is a problem shared by all forms of psychotherapy. This explains the gap between those who investigate psychotherapy and those who practice it, but do not find in EBM methods appropriate tools for assessing results. The implementation of EBM in medical practice in the 1990s was framed by the concept of 'managed care' and was linked to randomised clinical trial (RCT) as a methodological tool. It has been outlined that a major advantage of EBM is that it spreads a vast amount of information with the immediacy that current technology provides, and therefore, it contributes to the homogenisation of knowledge and standardisation of medical procedures. However, as pointed out by Thurin and colleagues (2007) and

Fischman and colleagues (2009), the drawback of EBM is that over time it turns out to be verificationist and leads to a limitation in the heuristic value of the research.

In 2012, we carried out a systematical review of RCT on group psychotherapy for psychosis from 1987 to 2011 (Tost, et al., 2010; Tost, Hernández and González de Chávez, 2012). The goal of this study was to explore the effectiveness of group psychotherapeutic treatments for people with psychosis according to EBM criteria. We later extended this study to include from 2012 to 2015. In both periods, we discovered that the aforementioned limitations of EBM were even greater in the case of group therapy. In this chapter, we discuss these flaws. In addition, we analyse the requirements of idiographic assessment methods, and in an attempt to propose other evaluation methods, we describe a novel approach of the Q-sort questionnaire of therapeutic factors proposed by Yalom (1985), based on a computerised gamification.

## A review of RCT on group therapy for psychosis

For our review (Tost, et al., 2010; Tost, Hernández and González de Chávez, 2012), a total number of 75 RCT were found. The sample includes 7,004 patients, predominantly males, with an average age of 37 years; and it covers 20 different countries, mainly Anglo-Saxon. In all cases, the diagnosis of participants was schizophrenia or schizo-affective disorder, according to the standard classification DSM (SCID)/CIE. In 76% of the trials, the origin and setting of the procedure were ambulatory.

The reviewed RCT studies were grounded in four main techniques: social skills training (SST), cognitive behaviour therapy (CBT), psychoeducational therapy (PE) and integrated psychological therapy (IPT). All of them were applied in group format. The average length of interventions was consistent with other systematic reviews (an average of 16 sessions); the shorter for CBT and the longer for SST (including booster sessions in the follow up).

Regarding the quality requirements of the RCT for psychotherapies, the conditions aimed at homogenising the experimental conditions to ensure the internal validity of the test were fulfilled in most reviewed trials. First, all trials used guidelines or a standardised intervention. Second, therapists were trained and supervised in most cases. Participant samples were homogeneous according to diagnosis criteria of current classifications with specific sub-profiles of decline, chronicity or presence of persistent auditory hallucinations for voice-oriented CBT.

For the assessment of the trial's methodological quality, we used the Jadad scale (Jadad, et al., 1996). This validated tool describes three indicators of quality design that reflect the internal validity of a trial and its bias probability: the randomised assignment method, the evaluators masking, and the attrition rate. Masking of assessors is the most neglected aspect of design in RCT literature (estimated outcomes inflation of 40%) and our analysis is consistent with this point. Reviewed CBT trials got the best scores on the Jadad scale, followed by SST, IPT and PE.

## Challenges for nomothetic RCT evaluations

With regard to the evaluated techniques, many trials combined two or more of the four abovementioned techniques, making it difficult to examine outcomes from a comparative point of view. For example, IPT was combined with several modules of SST, and CBT was integrated with SST. IPT is an 'integrated treatment' by itself that combines cognitive training, problem solving and social skills training.

Several questions need to be raised regarding the conditions of the RCT. First, the assumption that mental health problems can be solved in 16 or fewer sessions is not consistent with evidences for a significant psychotherapy dose-response relationship (see Shean, 2014). Second, the use of therapy guidelines biases research in favor of operationable therapies. Third, the requirement of trained and supervised therapists as a guarantee of fidelity to the technique, implicitly assumes that psychotherapy can be formulated as a standardised set of procedures applicable across individuals without significant variation in relation to therapists or patients (Shean, 2014). Fourth, the practice of patient selection based on uncomplicated DSM classification symptoms does not reflect the complexity of the clinical reality. Moreover, participants with the same diagnosis show different personality traits, attitudes, motivation towards the intervention, and capacities, all of which affect therapeutic results.

As already mentioned, CBT achieved the best scores in the Jadad scale, which is congruent with the facts that its context is well structured and generally shorter, with all variables controlled, and that it uses small samples. Does this mean that CBT shows a superior efficacy? As established in Wykes' CBT meta-analysis (Wykes, et al., 2008), and in later studies, it seems on the contrary: that the best design is associated with worst results, and poorer designs lead to inflated results. Indeed, Jauhar and colleagues (2014) criticise NICE for recommending the use of CBT in psychosis in spite of its small effect-size on all core symptoms and its worst results in comparison to other techniques if bias is considered.

Although all the interventions were delivered in groups, and techniques like PE and SST are generally designed for this format (whereas in CBT, the individual is prominent), the group context seems to be irrelevant in the description of the different techniques. However, Gabrovšek (2009) points out that above any technique, group therapy primarily relies on verbal communication, that the individual group member is the object of therapy, and that the group itself is the main therapeutic factor. None of the RCT devote attention to these postulates, which establish in essence the therapeutic strength of the group. So why is this type of format chosen in trials? Even if it can be supposed that cost-effective reasons underlie this option, this is nevertheless not explicitly stated.

Although RCT do not take into account the singular therapeutic ingredients of the group, it seems clear that these elements cannot be overlooked, and that not considering them calls into question the scientific process of RCT itself. This question is particularly evident in the choice of the trial control group. Treatment as Usual (TAU) or Waiting List (WL) are usually not recommended in current psychotherapy research for control groups because of obvious ethical considerations, and because they introduce a Hawthorne bias in results. Besides, the large variety of TAU related to the different healthcare system resources can also affect results. Moreover, evidence-based psychotherapies need to demonstrate benefits above what can be attributed to the non-specific effects of psychological interventions. Therefore, when a tested technique is compared with TAU/WL (60% of the reviewed RCT), the causal relationship between results and specific ingredients of the technique cannot be well established. However when using an active control group, as recommended by EBM, the lack of superiority in results of the tested technique can mean that the control intervention is at least as effective as the tested one, or that the shared (non-specific) ingredients running in the two groups lower the gap between the two interventions. Jauhar and colleagues (2014) point out that research may be flawed when the logic of placebo-controlled trials to psychotherapy is applied. Far from being unwanted complications that must be removed from trials, non-specific factors would be intrinsic elements of the trial without which nothing can be expected to happen in psychotherapy (Shean, 2014). Therefore, these factors need to be taken into account in all forms of psychotherapy research.

Although the different types of psychosocial treatment of schizophrenia focus on specific impairments, outcomes are not always linked to the treatment goal. SST focuses on the enhancement of social competency and social adaptation, but RCT assess secondary outcomes, such as relapses or psychotic symptoms reduction, which cannot be expected to be improved with this technique. Besides, although participants usually manage to replicate techniques trained in SST role play or in cognitive remediation exercises in IPT, the application and generalisation of these skills to daily functioning is not guaranteed. Being able to replicate trained skills is not as important as 'learning to learn', which depends on aspects such as autonomy, motivation or social competence.

Regarding CBT trials, global scales like PANSS (Positive and Negative Syndrome Scale) or BPRS (Brief Psychiatric Rating Scale) are hardly sensible to subtle changes produced by a specific intervention, which can probably explain its poor results. Regarding hallucination, CBT continues assessing changes on intensity or frequency of voices rather than on the belief, omnipotence and distress associated with them. Nevertheless, Chadwick and colleagues (2016) recently address this aspect in mindfulness CBT, and find that participants improved at post-intervention, with reduced depression symptoms and feeling less controlled by voices.

Some CBT achieve superior results on secondary assessments like quality of life, self esteem and patient satisfaction, as compared with primary outcomes, but seem to be nevertheless unaware of the possible link between these benefits and the impact of non-specific factors on the therapy. Finally, some questions remain unanswered, such as: What is understood by psychological change? Do therapy results promote a real change in life for patients? How much time and how much change is expected to be evaluable for efficacy?

Some forms of psychotherapy do not fit the requirements of the experimental frame of RCT. For instance, there were no trials of insight-oriented, supportive or discussion groups, perhaps because biological approaches tend to consider them as old forms of therapy, lacking in evidence-based support, and so used them only as control intervention. The following characteristics of psychotherapy do not harmonise with the experimental frame of RCT:

- *More flexibility:* less perfect for an experimental setup, but in return more adaptable to the real world.
- *Spontaneous inter-relational dynamics:* participants and therapists utilise this relationship as the motor for therapeutic change.
- *Lack of protocol or guidelines:* yet this does not mean that they are without a technique, frame or theoretical corpus.
- *Emphasis on more subjective and subtle changes:* more difficult to be measured with current scales, but with a high impact on the quality of life for patients.

As a matter of fact, none of the nine RCT that incorporate a supportive-discussion control group could demonstrate superior results of the tested intervention. Moreover, when supportive therapy was compared to CBT, it was found to have a greater specific impact on auditory hallucination. It can be supposed that the multiplicity of group communication promotes a cognitive decenterment in the patient.

## Towards idiographic evaluations

A change of trend in the assessment of intervention techniques in group therapy is currently happening, partly because of the modest effect-size in outcomes of RCT, and partly because experimental interventions are difficult to apply to the daily functioning of patients and are not always well accepted by them. Thus, the latest CBT trials are introducing 'psychodynamic reformulations' and more humanistic-oriented approaches. Third-wave psychological interventions, which have gained relevance in mental health services, are beginning to be applied to persons with psychosis, as reflected in the WELLFOCUS PPT pilot RCT of Schrank and colleagues (2016), and in the CBT mindfulness RCT of Chadwick and colleagues (2016). Recent trials emphasise qualitative parameters concerning the participant level of satisfaction, quality of life and well being, which historically have been considered as secondary improvement measures. Moreover, research has started to search for means of measuring concepts such as hope and change in insight. Ultimately, practitioners claim that further research on therapies must be described in terms of recovery-related changes rather than symptom reduction.

There is a growing interest for mediators and moderators of the group process, such as alliance, group cohesion and empathy, which are associated with improvements in real and perceived symptoms (see Norcross, Beutler and Levant, 2006;

Johnson, et al., 2008). Besides, some authors state that the therapeutic relationships in group contexts are essential for benefiting from any technique. Orfanos and colleagues (2015) emphasise that group psychotherapy can improve negative symptoms and social functioning deficits, and that the effect occurs across different treatments and appears to be non-specific. Finally, Chadwick and colleagues (2016) and Lecomte and colleagues (2014) describe Yalom's factor of 'universality' as the motor of change, and Leclerc and Lecomte (2012) state that for early CBT, the answer for efficacy lies in the group format.

Hence, it seems to be accepted that not all questions about psychotherapy's evaluation are easily answerable by quantitative methods, and that it becomes necessary to make an effort to translate and adapt the scientific procedures to qualitative methods in order to better understand the particularities of psychosocial interventions. Furthermore, qualitative research can be a rigorous and reliable method for judging effective practice. The challenge today for idiographic evaluation methods is to be able to:

- assess and spread the treatment outcomes, by combining results across studies and minimising bias of judgment;
- generalise results, which is an important problem for idiographic methods that usually take small samples and individual data;
- utilise a common language that could concern all theoretical approaches beyond supportive or exploratory orientations;
- design easy and attractive tools for researchers and participants to assess outcomes (in contrast to long and descriptive data gathering);
- return to patients the results they achieve, which is extremely valuable for them.

## The THT gamification: A novel approach for idiographic evaluation

Yalom (1985) designed a standardised Q-sort questionnaire to assess the therapeutic factors in group therapy. Q-methodology has been used in a wide variety of disciplines, and it is particularly useful when researchers wish to understand and describe the variety of *subjective* viewpoints on an issue from a individual–intrinsic perspective. Yalom's instrument consists of a forced-choice rank ordering of 60 items typed on cards. Twelve categories of curative factors are defined, each described by five cards. The test consists of placing the 60 cards into seven stacks labeled from least helpful to most helpful. The test scores each factor and determines which has got the highest score.

In spite of its usefulness, the test is long and arduous for both patients and researchers. In order to ease its administration, we have been working on a computerised gamification of this test for the evaluation of group therapy. The purpose of gamification is the application of game mechanics in non-game contexts to engage and motivate persons to achieve their goals. The result of this work is a computerised tool (THT gamification) with which patients complete the test in a fast and fun way. The tool computes automatically the therapeutic factor that has been most relevant for the patient, and it provides immediate feedback of this factor to the patient. We think that this 'return value' is valuable for the patient. In addition, we have associated a famous quote to each of the therapeutic factors that the test shows to the patient as a gift. The test stores the results in a file for their further analysis. The test is freely available at http://sgcreb.cs.upc.edu. It has been translated from English to Spanish and French. It is ready to be downloaded and installed following the instructions supplied on the webpage.

We are currently applying the THT with group therapy for psychotic patients, and we have seen that patients enjoy it and have a great expectation about their scores. We have noticed that they share their feedback with the other members of the group and discuss them. It seems that better understanding of how the group helps them to cope with their vulnerabilities, also aids them to take an active part in their progress.

## Conclusions

We have outlined the lack of trials on psychodynamic group psychotherapies, probably due to their difficulties to fulfill RCT criteria. This shortage is misunderstood as a lack of efficacy, and as a consequence, these therapeutic procedures are excluded from the empirically validated psychotherapies and, therefore, are not recommended in clinical guides.

RCT, which has been the basis of the validation of different treatments over the last decades, has failed to demonstrate consistent results for standardised interventions. In spite of their rigorous appearance, they present methodological deficiencies, and hence their results are called into question. In addition, they do not address the therapeutic process of change and the factors operating within the group that are, in the words of Yalom (1985); 'the actual mechanisms of effecting change in the patient that influence the processes of recovery among group therapy clients'. Moreover, RCT do not consider the values and preferences, as well as the understanding of effectiveness, from the participants' perspective, which are so important for psychotherapy research.

It is now accepted that psychotherapy research cannot be equal to biomedical research methods, and that alternative idiographic approaches should be explored. We hope that the THT gamified Yalom's Q-sort can be useful for qualitative research on therapeutic factors for the group, because it provides a database of outcomes across researchers and contributes to the involvement of patients in an interactive process of assessing results.

## References

Chadwick, P., Strauss, C., Jones A-M., Kingdon, D., et al. (2016) Group mindfulness-based intervention for distressing voices: A pragmatic randomised controlled trial. *Schizophrenia Research,* 175(1–3), 168–173.

Chazan, R. (2001) *The Group as Therapist*. London: Jessica Kingsley.

Fischman, G., Advenier, F., Baruch, C., Brusset, B., et al. (2009). *L'Évaluation des Psychothérapies et de la Psychanalyse: Fondements et enjeux* [*Evaluation of Psychotherapies and Psychoanalysis: Foundations and issues*]. Paris: Edition Masson.

Gabrovšek, V. (2009) In-patient group therapy of patients with schizophrenia. *Psychiatria Danubina*, 21(1), 67–72.

González de Chávez, M. (2008) 'Psicoterapia de grupo y esquizofrenia' ['Group psychotherapy and schizophrenia'] in: Y.O. Alanen, M. González de Chávez, A-L.S. Silver and B. Martindale (Eds), *Abordajes Psicoterapéuticos de las Psicosis Esquizofrénicas* [*Psychotherapeutic Approaches to Schizophrenic Psychoses*]. Madrid: Fundación para la Investigación y Tratamiento de la Esquizofrenia y otras Psicosis.

Jadad, A.R., Moore, R.A., Carroll, D., Jenkinson, C., et al. (1996) Assessing the quality of reports of randomized clinical trials: Is blinding necessary? *Controlled Clinical Trials*, 17(1), 1–12.

Jauhar, S., McKenna, P.J., Radua, J., Fung, E., et al. (2014) Cognitive–behavioural therapy for the symptoms of schizophrenia: Systematic review and meta-analysis with examination of potential bias. *The British Journal of Psychiatry*, 204(1), 20–29.

Johnson, D.P., Penn, D.L., Bauer, D.J., Meyer, P., et al. (2008) Predictors of the therapeutic alliance in group therapy for individuals with treatment-resistant auditory hallucinations. *British Journal of Clinical Psychology*, 47(2), 171–184.

Kanas, N. (1986) Group psychotherapy with schizophrenics: A review of controlled studies. *International Journal of Group Psychotherapy*, 36(3), 339–351.

Leclerc, C. and Lecomte, T. (2012) TCC pour premiers épisodes de psychose: Pourquoi la thérapie de groupe obtient les meilleurs résultats? [CBT for first episode of psychosis: Why does group therapy offer better results?] *Journal de Thérapie Comportementale et Cognitive*, 22(3), 104–110.

Lecomte, T., Leclerc, C., Wykes, T., Nicole, L., et al. (2014) Understanding process in group cognitive behaviour therapy for psychosis. *Psychology and Pscychotherapy*, 88(2), 163–177.

Norcross, J.C., Beutler, L.E. and Levant, R.F. (2006) *Evidence-Based Practices in Mental Health: Debate and dialogue on the fundamental questions*. Washington: American Psychological Association.

Orfanos, S., Banks, C. and Priebe, S. (2015) Are group psychotherapeutic treatments effective for patients with schizophrenia? A systematic review and meta-analysis. *Psychotherapy and Psychosomatics*, 84(4), 241–249.

Schrank, B., Brownell, T., Jakaite, Z., Larkin, C., et al. (2016) Evaluation of a positive psychotherapy group intervention for people with psychosis: Pilot randomized controlled trial. *Epidemiology and Psychiatric Sciences*, 25(3), 235–246.

Shean, G. (2014) Limitations of randomized control designs in psychotherapy research. *Advances in Psychiatry*, 2014, ID 561452.

Thurin, J-M., Thurin, M., Lapeyronnie, B. and Briffault, X. (2007) *Évaluer les Psychotherapies: Méthodes et pratiques* [*Evaluate Psychotherapies: Methods and Practices*]. Paris: Dunod.

Tost, L., Hernández, C.B. and González de Chávez, M. (2012) 'Psicoterapia de grupo en la esquizofrenia durante los últimos 25 años. Una revisión basada en la evidencia' ['Group psychotherapy for schizophrenia during the last 25 years: An evidence-based review'] (pp. 305–359) in M. González de Chávez (Ed), *25 Años de Psicoterapia de Grupo en las*

*Psicosis* [*25 Years of Group Psychotherapy of Psychosis*]. Madrid: Fundación para la Investigación y Tratamiento de la Esquizofrenia y otras Psicosis.

Tost, L., Hernández, C., Rodrígues, F., Perestelo, L., et al. (2010) *Psicoterapia de grupo como técnica terapéutica en personas con esquizofrenia* [*Group psychotherapies as a therapeutic technique in people with schizophrenia*]. SESCS No. 2007/13. Madrid: Ministerio de Ciencia e Innovación.

Urlić, I. (2010) The group psychodynamic psychotherapy approach to patients with psychosis. *Psychiatria Danubina,* 22(1), 10–14.

Wykes, T., Steel, C., Everitt, B. and Tarrier, N. (2008) Cognitive behavior therapy for schizophrenia: Effect sizes, clinical models, and methodological rigor. *Schizophrenia Bulletin,* 34(3), 523–537.

Yalom, I. (1985) *The Theory and Practice of Group Psychotherapy,* 3rd edition. New York: Basic Books.

# Chapter 3

# Therapeutic factors in group psychotherapy for patients diagnosed with psychosis

*Ignacio García Cabeza*

## Introduction

Yalom (1970) defines group therapy factors as therapeutic action mechanisms that act by favouring change and that contribute to the therapeutic process inherent in group interaction or dynamics. They are not directly associated to the action of the therapist. They are basic or elemental components of the phenomenon of therapeutic change derived from the group matrix.

The study of group therapy factors began in the mid-1950s when Corsini and Rosenberg (1955) reviewed more than 300 articles on group psychotherapy, with the goal of ordering and classifying the essential mechanisms for therapeutic success. After their study, different classifications were recognised (see Table 3.1).

The Yalom study is of special interest. One reason is because it develops a Q-sort questionnaire that permits the systematic study and analysis of the group therapy factors. In addition, it is also of interest due to the theoretical contributions made by the author to group therapy as a whole. Yalom abandoned the group-analytic postulates and began to stress the importance of the interpersonal sphere. In fact, he incorporated two forms of interpersonal learning within the group therapy factors: input (that which is mainly acquired through other group members) and output (where the subject attempts to develop more adaptive methods of relating with others) (Yalom, 1985).

Yalom described 12 therapeutic factors (see Table 3.1), but he states that they must be considered as arbitrary constructs that are not independent and that do not occur or act separately. While these factors operate in all types of group, how they act greatly differs according to variables such as type of group, type of participation in the group and the point in time (Yalom and Leszcz, 2005). Even more importantly, although therapeutic factors are key elements in the process of group change, they should be integrated together with other specific elements of the group therapy, such as mirroring and the context, because they are all responsible elements of the therapeutic process that confer a specific uniqueness to the group and have great therapeutic value (González de Chávez, 2008).

*Table 3.1* Principal classifications of the group therapeutic factors

| | | |
|---|---|---|
| Corsini and Rosenberg (1955) | 3 categories, 9 factors | *Intellectual:* universality, intellectualisation and spectator therapy<br>*Emotional:* acceptance, altruism and transference<br>*Behavioral:* reality testing, interaction and ventilation |
| Yalom (1985) | 12 factors (*) | Altruism, cohesion, universality, interpersonal learning input, interpersonal learning output, guidance, catharsis, identification, family re-enactment, understanding, hope and existential factors |
| Bloch and Crouch (1985) | 10 factors | Self-understanding, interaction, cohesion, self-disclosure, catharsis, guidance, universality, altruism, vicarious learning and installation of hope |
| MacKenzie (1990) | 4 categories, 12 factors | *Support:* hope, acceptance, universality and altruism<br>*Self-disclosure:* self-disclosure and catharsis<br>*Learning from other members of the group:* modelling, vicarious learning, guidance and education<br>*Psychological work:* self-understanding and interpersonal learning |
| Dierick and Lietaer (2008) | 3 hierchical levels and 2 dimensions | 3 levels of abstraction (conscious, pre-conscious and unconscious), with seven principles scales (cohesion, interactional confirmation, cathartic self-disclosure, self-insight and progress, observational experiences, obtaining of directives and interactional confrontation), and two dimensions (relational climate and psychological work) |

Notes
(*) Yalom initially described nine factors (Yalom, 1970), to which he subsequently added three more: installation of hope, guidance and existential factors.

## Therapeutic factors in group psychotherapy

For didactic purposes, we will use the MacKenzie classification (1990) to describe the group therapy factors. He developed an operational and practical classification, with four general groups: support factors, self-disclosure, learning from other members of the group and psychological work (see Table 3.1).

Beginning with **support factors**, *instillation of hope* acts in the initial moments by favouring group survival and continuity of its members. In addition, seeing how other patients have overcome similar situations favours the enthusiasm and motivation of the others. Its importance increases when dealing with patients with chronic diseases (Yalom and Leszcz, 2005). *Universality* permits patients to abandon their singularity. They come to the group considering that they are the only ones who have certain problems or fears, fantasies, impulses and thoughts, or who have suffered or undergone unacceptable situations. The simple fact of hearing that others have experiences and problems similar to theirs is a relief.

In groups of patients with psychosis, desingularisation allows them to stop feeling they are the only ones who experience unique realities and identities. Together with agreed-on validation of these experiences, the patient acquires an awareness of suffering a mental disorder (González de Chávez, Cabeza and Fraile, 1999). In relation to the *altruism* factor, the patients not only benefit by the reciprocal fact of giving and receiving, but also by the intrinsic and gratifying utility entailed in offering something to others; a differential element of group therapies versus individual interventions. The patients offer support, consolation and suggestions. The last support factor is *acceptance,* with a similar meaning to the cohesion of Yalom (1985); see below. These factors are valued, above all, in inpatients' groups (Mushet, Whalan and Power, 1989).

All these factors and those described further below are linked with **self-disclosure**, which is even better if it is accompanied by cognitive learning (learning to communicate feelings) and emotional expression, in the form of *catharsis*. It is not easy for the patients in whom isolation is generally a common problem to find a place where they can speak and express feelings (Kanas and Barr, 1982).

Included within the **learning factors** are features that go from information (whether given by the therapist or provided by other patients) to socialisation techniques (such as imitation, modelling or vicarious learning). *Education* or *didactic information* is a key element in psychoeducational groups for many somatic and mental diseases, including schizophrenia, and it has demonstrated certain efficacy in the prevention of relapses (Xia, Merinder and Belgamwar, 2011). In addition, education is used in several ways in group psychotherapy to: transfer information, structure the group, explain the process of the disease, alter thinking patterns and, more importantly, to correct mistaken ideas regarding the disease (Yalom and Leszcz, 2005). Another form of information is *advice* or direct and shared guidance between patients. This appears systematically in the first phases of interactive groups, although its greatest value is generally the fact of 'giving', since it implies mutual interest and concern, more than the advice itself (Yalom, 1970). It acquires added value in groups of psychotics oriented towards problem-solving or communication skills. The passive factors of learning, *imitation, identification,* or *vicarious learning* are probably understated and are those least rated in most studies. However, the patients may obtain important benefits that they do not always perceive when they observe how others cope with similar problems, above all in the initial stages of the group. This could become the initiation of experiencing new forms of relationships and actions that could imply future and deeper changes (Yalom and Leszcz, 2005; González de Chávez, 2008).

Self-understanding and interpersonal learning are included within the **psychological work factors**. In outpatient groups, the *self-understanding* factor is always one of the most valued (Butler and Fuhriman, 1980, 1983; Bloch and Reibstein, 1980; Hobbs, et al., 1989; Vlastelica, Urlić and Pavlović, 2001). However, knowledge acquisition cannot be understood within the groups without the participation of *interpersonal learning*. The patients initially acquire insight through the image of themselves that others return to them. This is followed by a deeper process of understanding their behaviour patterns, until they come to understand why they do what they do and they behave as they do, in order to perhaps finally understand how they have reached this point (Yalom and Leszcz, 2005). During the group process, the image and identity of each group member is continually questioned, made more flexible, shaped and defined. This occurs both by that which the patients observe in themselves and learn from others, as well as through the feedback received from the others, all of which shape a new identity and a new vision of oneself (González de Chávez and Capilla, 1993a, 1993b).

Finally, we will make some comments on a factor that was essential for Yalom and was not included in the MacKenzie classification: *cohesion*. This describes the result of all forces that act on the members of the group to remain in it, and it is similar to the therapeutic relationship within individual psychotherapy (Yalom, 1985). The definition *per se* may be why some authors have not included it within the therapeutic factors, but rather have considered cohesiveness as a necessary precondition. It is not considered as a single construct, but rather as a sum of elements included within the therapeutic factors, which would work in mutual re-inforcement (MacKenzie, 1990), providing a safe climate that facilitates interaction in the group (Kanas, 1996).

## Therapeutic factors in groups of patients with diagnosis of psychoses

There are only a few studies on therapeutic factors in groups of psychotic patients. Furthermore, many of these have been performed with groups that are heterogeneous in their diagnoses and with patients in hospitalisation units. Maxmen and Hanover (1973) found that the most valued therapeutic factors (20% schizophrenia diagnosis) were instillation of hope, cohesion, altruism and universality. Leszcz and colleagues (1985) suggested that the favoured therapeutic factors depend on the level of ego functioning. Support factors and guidance have more value in chronic psychosis inpatients with low ego functioning. With a similar approach, Kahn and colleagues (1986) concluded that instillation of hope is the most valued factor among patients with a low ego-functioning level. Standing out among the studies performed in the outpatient setting, the study of Butler and Fuhriman (1980), in a day hospital with a predominance of psychotic patients, found that cohesion, identification and family re-enactment were rated as the most valued factors. An overview of the studies with homogeneous groups of psychotic patients is shown in Table 3.2.

Kanas and colleagues studied two homogeneous groups of schizophrenic patients, these being inpatients and a short-duration outpatients group. Both gave priority to having a place in which to interact with others, compare psychotic experiences and express feelings (as opposed to valuing insight and obtaining advice). Factors such as altruism or universality occupy the second and fourth place

Table 3.2 Investigations on therapeutic factors with homogenous groups of psychotic patients

| Study | Most valued factor | Least valued factor | Significant differences |
|---|---|---|---|
| Kanas and Barr (1982) Inpatient groups | A place to express emotions | Guidance/advice | |
| Kanas, Stewart and Habey (1988) Outpatient groups | Trust in others | Guidance/advice | |
| Rico and Sunyer (2001) Outpatient groups | Interpersonal learning output | Identification | Patients with better prognosis give more value to self-understanding, and those with worse prognosis value hope |
| González de Chávez, et al. (2000) Groups of psychotic patients: inpatients versus outpatients | Inpatient: hope Outpatient: hope | Inpatient: identification Outpatient: identification | Outpatients give significantly more value to self-understanding and less value to cohesion |
| García Cabeza and González de Chávez (2009) Psychotic outpatient groups according to degree of insight | Hope, independently of degree of insight | Identification, independently of degree of insight | Patients with more insight give significantly more value to self- understanding |
| García Cabeza, et al. (2011) Inpatient groups: psychosis versus affective | Psychosis: hope Affective: hope | Psychosis: identification Affective: identification | |
| Outpatient groups: schizophrenia versus bipolar | Psychosis: hope Bipolar: hope | Psychosis: identification Bipolar: identification | |
| Outpatient groups: patients versus therapists | Patients: self-understanding Therapists: self-understanding | Patients: identification Therapists: guidance | Therapists give significantly more value to self-understanding and less value to cohesion and guidance |

in the assessment of the hospitalised patients, while they are third and fourth in the outpatients (Kanas and Barr, 1982; Kanas, Stewart and Habey, 1988). Kanas also notes the importance of cohesion as an element having great therapeutic value in this type of group (Kanas, 1996).

Rico and Sunyer (2001) found that the factors that were most highly valued in groups of psychotic outpatients were cohesion and interpersonal learning output. He found that instillation of hope was highly rated among patients with worse prognosis, and self-understanding among those with a better prognosis.

Our team has performed five investigations on therapeutic factors in group therapy in which at least one of the groups studied was homogenously formed by psychotic patients in the spectrum of schizophrenia. In the first study, we compared in- and outpatients groups of psychotic patients. The three therapeutic factors considered as most useful for the inpatients were hope, cohesion and altruism. For the outpatients these were hope, self-understanding and universality. The only statistically significant differences were found in the self-understanding factor (most valued in the outpatient group) and cohesion (with greater scores by hospitalised patients) (González de Chávez, et al., 2000). The second study compared groups of psychotic outpatients in accordance with their grade of insight. Regardless of the grade of insight, the most valued factor was instillation of hope and the least rated was identification. Only the self-understanding factor varied significantly based on the degree of insight; self-understanding was valued much more by those patients who achieved greater insight (García Cabeza and González de Chávez, 2009).

In our last publication, we included three new studies (García Cabeza, et al., 2011). In the first, two inpatients groups (affective versus psychosis) were compared. There was practically total agreement for the results regarding the best-valued factors (hope, altruism, interpersonal learning output and cohesion) and the least-valued factors (identification, interpersonal learning input, family re-enactment and guidance). In the second study, we compared two outpatient groups (bipolar versus schizophrenia). The results in the highest rated factors (instillation of hope, altruism and guidance) were the same. In the last research, we compared the ratings of the factors given by the patients, all of whom had a diagnosis of schizophrenia, as well as the evaluation by the therapists and co-therapists of these groups. Significant differences were observed in the evaluation of the guidance factors; cohesion and guidance factors were less valued by the therapists, and self-understanding more highly valued.

## Therapeutic factors in our clinical practice

From these studies, we can conclude that the most valued factors in groups of patients with psychosis are those which involve support (in fact, installation of hope is the most valued factor in almost all of the studies described). Factors related with psychological work (the most valued in outpatient groups) are only given priority in long-duration groups, patients with high ego functioning (Leszcz,

Yalom and Nordem, 1985), better prognosis (Rico and Sunyer, 2001), or a higher degree of insight (García Cabeza and González de Chávez, 2009).

The support factors work together to promote the climate or therapeutic alliance and to favour cohesion. As we have already said, hope favours attendance and strengthens optimism. Universality helps the patient to decrease isolation and to relieve the feeling of uniqueness by sharing similar experiences, and so allows them to initiate a process of forming a new self-concept. Altruism offers the possibility to help others and thus learn about one's own feelings and positive aspects. These elements are dominant in the first stages of the groups, but they also play an important role during the therapeutic process as they open the way to interpersonal learning and self-understanding factors (Liberman, 1983; Yalom, 1985; Bloch and Crouch, 1985), which helps the patients to overcome their negative symptoms, isolation and affective poverty.

Self-understanding and universality allow identifications, self-disclosures, help and validations on transferences or significant relations, with the possibility of interpersonal learning. The group context also offers cognitive decentralisation and corrections to egocentrism. Insight on the characteristics of the vulnerable identity and psychotic defenses, first acted out in the group, can then be recognised and perhaps modified later on. Thus, self-understanding cannot be understood without the interaction with others – factors such as interpersonal learning input and output. Self-knowledge is largely obtained through interpersonal understanding. As we have seen, these become two inseparable aspects in the mechanism of change, both regarding development of the personality of the subject as well as correction of psychopathological problems (Anthony, 1971; González de Chávez and Capilla, 1993a, 1993b). Even more, none of this would be possible without the self-disclosure and catharsis factors; preconditions for self-understanding and learning (Bloch and Crouch, 1985; Yalom, 1985). Passive learning factors, although generally modestly valued, may even be a source of stimulation for the most passive patients, promoting identifications and imitation and becoming an important element of change in psychoeducational and support groups (González de Chávez, 2008).

In summary, the group should be the therapeutic tool *per se*. Its specific and differential characteristics (context, mirroring and the therapeutic factors) should be understood as a whole that acts simultaneously and synergically, encouraging understanding and change in the patient. Initially, through desingularisation and agreed-on validation of the reality, the patient can acquire awareness that they have a mental disorder. Subsequently, through self-reflection and feedback from others, the patient may discover his/her most hidden and unconscious parts, vulnerabilities and defense mechanisms, and may be able to provide meaning to his/her psychotic experiences. Finally, it may be possible for those patients who have greater capacity of insight, and always with the help of the entire group, to be able to integrate their psychosis and give meaning to their psychosis within their biographic experience (González de Chávez, 2012).

## Clinical vignette 3.1

Patient H was in his thirties when he was first admitted to hospital. His father was hospitalised and while he was visiting him, he began to verbalise that his father was dead and that the world was going to end. He lived with his mother and was the youngest of three siblings. His father suffered dementia associated with Parkinson's disease and died shortly after H's first admission.

The parents of H separated while he was an adolescent. The characters of both parents differed greatly. His mother was very concerned about her family and, in general, quite obsessive. The life of his father was quite bohemian and he had been unfaithful several times before he initiated a new relationship and proposed the definitive separation. His father moved to a foreign country and promised H that he would take him with him. This never occurred. H always blamed his mother for his father's leaving: in fact, he idealised his father and his new wife, a bohemian and artist. H referred to the new wife as 'mother' and to his birth mother as 'biological mother'. During his entire adolescence, reproaches between mother and son were frequent. H even often ate alone in his room – 'even her cough bothered me'. Coinciding with his father's return, H dropped out of school in the University Orientation Course and began to work with his father in publicity. He always worked without a contract, even though all of his family recognised his value (in fact, he had some success composing electronic music in the 1980s).

A loner and distrustful, H had a pessimistic view of the world and sexual identity problems. He only had one relationship with a girl, with whom he had an intense friendship, and who committed suicide shortly before his father was hospitalised. Even though they no longer had a stable relationship, they had promised each other to 'spend their whole lives together'. He also had few social relationships, and those that he did have were almost always associated with his interests (music, drawing, etc.). All of these relationships disappeared over the years, generally because they did not share his view of the world.

Shortly after he was discharged from hospital, H abandoned treatment and his withdrawal intensified. He focused exclusively on internet chatting and began to feel progressively that all his activities were controlled through the computer, and that he was being watched. Psychotic experiences having apocalyptic content progressively began to appear. Two years later, he was re-admitted.

After this admission, it was decided to include H in group therapy. The support he received in the first group sessions made it possible for him to maintain the treatment. Furthermore, some significant results could be seen from his first sessions. In one of them, when he arrived he was very anxious, trying to speak with his psychiatrist. Since it was time for the group to begin and he said he did not want to speak in the group, the interview was postponed. During the session, H did not speak. However, he heard the paranoid interpretations and constructions of delusions of another patient. When he left the session, H was calm and said that he could wait until the next session, where he spoke, with the help of the group, about interpretations that he had been able to control. This highlights that desingularisation and emerging from perceptive egocentism favour control of psychotic experiences and the acquisition of some awareness of mental disorder that is the first step towards acquiring insight.

Later on, with the help of other group members, H began to understand some of the meanings of his psychoses and the role played by the death of his father, with whom he not only had shared an affective relationship but also an affective and economical dependence. Another member of the group stated: *You suffered a personal crisis; your girlfriend committed suicide, your father died and you transferred your personal crisis to a world crisis.*

Over time, H has explored deeper into the knowledge of his psychoses, as well as his interpersonal problems, and has recognised the losses (abandoned by his father, betrayed by his girlfriend, etc.) as key elements in his isolation and distrustfulness when establishing interpersonal relations. Another member of the group stated: *I think that it is because of everything that has occurred to you during your lifetime. This will continue to occur forever if you do not solve this. When you have the tools, you will be able to analyse and understand it . . . to know the tools is to know why certain things are happening to you.*

After several years of therapy and other crises that did not require admissions or increased antipsychotic doses, H has been able to admit his homosexuality and maintain several relationships with a partner. He has recovered friends from the better times of his life when he wrote music and has even carried out business with electronic music devices through the internet. He has also begun to draw again, although not professionally. He has several friendships and is planning on becoming independent from his mother.

*Comment:* As has already been stated, the factors that initially act in group therapies are those of support, in this case mainly hope and universality, that allow patients to feel welcome, to feel listened to and understood, that would favour the patient's adherence. Later, as group cohesion increases and through disclosure, other factors begin to act, such as learning, which is initially passive and then interpersonal, as well as the understanding of internal and external factors that may affect the development of the psychosis. These factors, some of them specific to group therapy (universality, interpersonal learning, etc.) have a unique therapeutic potential that makes the group a singular and especially effective element in the treatment of patients with psychosis.

## References

Anthony, E.J. (1971) 'Comparison between individual and group psychotherapy' (pp. 104–117) in H. Kaplan and B. Saddock (Eds), *Comprehensive Group Psychotherapy*, 1st edition. Baltimore: Williams & Wilkins.

Bloch, S. and Crouch, E. (1985) *Therapeutic Factors in Group Psychotherapy.* Oxford: Oxford University Press.

Bloch, S., Crouch, E. and Reibstein, J. (1981) Therapeutic factors in group psychotherapy. *Archives of General Psychiatry*, 38, 519–526.

Bloch, S. and Reibstein, J. (1980) Perceptions by patients and therapists of therapeutic factors in group psychotherapy. *The British Journal of Psychiatry*, 137, 274–278.

Butler, T. and Fuhriman, A. (1980) Patients' perspective on the curative process: A comparison of day treatment and outpatients psychotherapy groups. *Small Group Behaviour*, 11, 371–388.

Butler, T. and Fuhriman, A. (1983) Level of functioning and length of time in treatment variables influencing patients' therapeutic experience in group psychotherapy. *International Journal of Group Psychotherapy*, 33, 189–205.

Corsini, R.J. and Rosenberg, B. (1955) Mechanisms of group psychotherapy: Processes and dynamics. *Journal of Abnormal Social Psychology*, 51, 406–411.

Dierick, P. and Lietaer, G. (2008) Client perception of therapeutic factors in group psychotherapy and growth groups: An empirically-based hierarchical model. *International Journal of Group Psychotherapy*, 58(2), 203–230.

García Cabeza, I., Ducajú, M., Gutiérrez, M. and González de Chávez, M. (2011) Therapeutic factors in group of patients with psychosis. *Group Analysis*, 4, 419–436.

García Cabeza, I. and González de Chávez, M. (2009) Insight and therapeutic factors in group psychotherapy for schizophrenic outpatients. *Psychosis*, 1, 134–144.

González de Chávez, M. (2008) 'Terapia de grupo y esquizofrenia' ['Group therapy and schizophrenia'] (pp: 293–313) in: Y.O. Alanen, M. González de Chávez, A-L.S. Silver and B. Martindale (Eds), *Abordajes Psicoterapéuticos de las Psicosis Esquizofrénicas* [*Psychotherapeutic Apporaches to Schizophrenic Psychoses*]. Madrid: Fundación para la Investigación y Tratamiento de la Esquizofrenia y otras Psicosis.

González de Chávez, M. (2012) *25 Años de Psicoterapia de Grupo en la Psicosis* [*25 Years of Group Psychotherapy of Psychosis*]. Madrid: Fundación para la Investigación y Tratamiento de la Esquizofrenia y otras Psicosis.

González de Chávez, M. and Capilla, T. (1993a) Autoconocimiento y reacciones especulares en psicoterapia de grupo con pacientes esquizofrénicos (I) [Insight and mirroring in group psychotherapy with schizophrenic patients 1]. Madrid: *Revista de la Asociación Española de Neuropsiquiatría*, 13(44), 29–34.

González de Chávez, M. and Capilla, T. (1993b) Autoconocimiento y reacciones especulares en psicoterapia de grupo con pacientes esquizofrénicos (II) [Insight and mirroring in group psychotherapy with schizophrenic patients 2]. Madrid: *Revista de la Asociación Española de Neuropsiquiatría,* 13(45), 103–112.

González de Chávez, M., García Cabeza, I. and Fraile, J.C. (1999) Dos grupos psicoterapéuticos de pacientes esquizofrénicos: Hospitalizados y ambulatorios [Two psychotherapeutic groups of schizophrenic patients: Inpatient and outpatient]. *Revista de la Asociación Española de Neuropsiquiatría,* 19(72), 573–586.

González de Chávez, M., Gutiérrez, M., Ducajú, M. and Fraile, J.C. (2000) Comparative study of the therapeutic factors of group therapy in schizophrenic inpatients and outpatients. *Group Analysis,* 33, 251–264.

Hobbs, M., Birtchnell, S., Harte, A. and Lacey, H. (1989) Therapeutic factors in short-term group therapy for women with bulimia. *International Journal of Eating Disorders,* 8, 623–633.

Kahn, E., Webster, P.B. and Storck, M. (1986). Curative factors in two types of inpatient psychotherapy groups. *International Journal of Group Psychotherapy,* 36, 579–585.

Kanas, N. (1996). *Group Therapy for Schizophrenic Patients.* Clinical practice series, No. 39. Arlington, VA: American Psychiatric Association.

Kanas, N. and Barr, M.A. (1982) Short-term homogeneous group therapy for schizophrenia inpatients: A questionnaire evaluation. *Group,* 6(4), 32–38.

Kanas, N., Stewart, P. and Habey, K. (1988) Content and outcome in a short-term therapy group for schizophrenic outpatients. *Hospital and Community Psychiatry,* 39, 437–439.

Kapur, R., Miller, K. and Mitchell, G. (1988) Therapeutic factors within inpatients and outpatients psychotherapy groups. *The British Journal of Psychiatry,* 152, 229–233.

Lese, K.P. and MacNair-Semands, R.R. (2000) The therapeutic Factors Inventory: Development of a scale. *Group,* 24, 303–317.

Leszcz, M., Yalom, I.D. and Nordem, M. (1985) The value of inpatient group psychotherapy: Patient's perception. *International Journal of Group Psychotherapy,* 35, 41–433.

Liberman, M.A. (1983) 'Comparative analyses of change mechanisms in groups' in R.R. Dies and K.R. MacKenzie (Eds), *Advances in Group Psychotherapy.* New York: International University Press.

MacKenzie, K.R. (1990) *Introduction to Time-Limited Group Psychotherapy,* 1st edition. Washington: American Psychiatric Press.

Maxmen, J.S. and Hanover, M.D. (1973) Group therapy as viewed by hospitalized patients. *Archives of General Psychiatry,* 28, 404–408.

McGlashan, T.H. (1994) What has become of the psychotherapy of schizophrenia? *Acta Psychiatrica Scandinavica,* 90 (supl. 384), 147–152.

Mushet, G.L., Whalan, G.S. and Power, R. (1989) In-patients' views of the helpful aspects of group psychotherapy impact of therapeutic style and treatment setting. *British Journal of Medical Psychology,* 2, 135–141.

Rico, L. and Sunyer, M. (2001) Análisis comparativo de los factores terapéuticos grupales en la esquizofrenia (II): Resultados y discusión [Comparative analysis of group therapeutic factors in schizophrenia. Part II. Results and discussion]. *Psiquis,* 22(2), 57–72.

Vlastelica, M., Urlić, I. and Pavlović, S. (2001) The assessment of the analytic group treatment efficiency according to Yalom's classification. *Collegium Antropologicum,* 25, 227–237.

Xia, J., Merinder, L.B. and Belgamwar, M.R. (2011) Psychoeducation for schizophrenia. *The Cochrane Database of Systematic Reviews*, 15(6), CD002831.

Yalom, I. (1970) *The Theory and Practice of Group Psychotherapy*, 1st edition. New York: Basic Books.

Yalom, I. (1985) *The Theory and Practice of Group Psychotherapy*, 3rd edition. New York: Basic Books.

Yalom, I. and Leszcz, M. (2005) *The Theory and Practice of Group Psychotherapy*, 5th edition. New York: Basic Books.

Chapter 4

# Creation of a therapy group for persons with psychotic experiences

*Manuel González de Chávez*

In this chapter, we will explain the main aspects to consider when we intend to create a therapy group for persons with psychotic experiences. These include those that arise from the care organisation and institutional functioning where the group will be located, and those related to the evaluation and initial selection of the patients for a newly created group or for the inclusion of new patients in an already established group that functions on a regular basis.

## Mental health organisation

The possibilities for creating a therapy group for persons with psychotic disorders are very diverse. However, they largely depend on the care context and institutions where the group is conducted, on the group's team of therapists, the approaches or usual understanding of the disorders these patients suffer, and on the proposed group therapeutic objectives and tasks.

The acute units of general hospitals; mental health care centres, hospitals or day centres; residential centres or rehabilitation units; therapeutic communities; and, in general, any section of the mental health care service organisation that attends psychotic persons, do so for persons with differentiated characteristics. Therefore, the therapeutic groups that can be created in them should have specific objectives and tasks, in accordance with the care demands and general functions of the specific institution where the therapy groups may be located. Even so, based on the training and points of views of the members of the therapeutic teams interested in creating these groups, in all these institutions it is possible to create groups that have different approaches and objectives, and with varied theoretical perspectives, as cognitive–behavioural, dynamic, interpersonal, existential and problem-solving groups, to name a few. Furthermore, the group can be conducted with practical undertakings and very diverse formats in terms of size, composition and duration.

However, we must keep in mind that the viability of the therapy groups, their continuity over time and the regular channelling and volume of patients, is sufficient for the group to be therapeutic. This will always depend on the concordance of the groups created with the usual demands of the care service where the group will be located. Creation of a therapy group should always be oriented towards the needs of the patients of the institution and not on the preferences or satisfactions of the professionals who can or want to create such a therapy group.

In addition, the group cannot be an isolated therapeutic cell within the healthcare and social organisation. It can only function when working together as a whole with the care activities and programmes that care for the patient before, during and after the group therapy. The groups can only survive and have meaning within this combination. We cannot expect a therapy group to be a single and global treatment by itself of patients with psychotic experiences.

## The institutional functioning

It is of utmost importance to understand and have an impact on the functioning of the institution in which a psychotherapy group is going to be created. This is in regard to: the facilities (including group rooms, offices, waiting rooms or administrative support); the necessary choosing, motivation and training of the group therapists; and also the full collaboration of the institution if therapy groups are to be considered attractive and an asset to the centre. The institution needs to provide the group with a regular flow of patients that can benefit from them, progressing and remaining in the group over time.

This involvement of the institution with group therapies is valid for both public centres and private practices. There are institutions that have sophisticated channelling and evaluation systems of the patients who are candidates for group therapy (Brown, 1991). There is also evidence that the care organisation services headed by professionals with group therapy experience create more therapy groups, evaluating and channelling more patients to them as well as reducing the number of drop-outs in the groups. The opposite occurs when the centre management has no interest in group therapies (Yalom, 1966, 1983).

However, along with the administrative power of the professionals, teaching and training the nursing staff and all the healthcare personnel about group dynamics and the basic foundations of group therapy and its therapeutic objectives is also important, especially if the institution has inpatients (Battegay, 1971). The institution *per se* should ensure that all the professionals are trained, especially regarding the knowledge and skill of the therapists who lead the groups of these patients. This task must be adequately encouraged in relationship to the performance of the other common clinical tasks and should not be an extra burden for the group therapists. Sometimes, a certain level of schedule flexibility becomes necessary; for example, to facilitate patient attendance to outpatient groups or when these groups are conducted outside of the work schedule of the centre staff.

The characteristics of the group therapist are key to its functioning, beginning with its creation and continuing during the entire therapeutic process (Dies, 1994). In groups dedicated to persons with psychotic experiences, the commitment, effort, motivation and empathy of the therapists with these patients are essential (Urlić, 1999). Grandiose, narcissist and messianic therapists have no place here. The task is slow, often modest in achievements, sometimes difficult to follow and understand, with many personal and biographical limitations in the group members, and blockages, impasses and frustrations are common in the therapeutic progress. The therapist must have sufficient sensitivity, patience and realism to always lead the group, differentiating his/her professional identity from the changing tides of the group dynamics, which sometimes is submerged in painful psychotic experiences by some members who seem to carry the entire group into an insurmountable collapse. The therapist must know how to get the group back on its feet, without fantasies, or voluntarisms, but rather with hope and pragmatism.

A therapy group with psychotic patients, and even more so with patients in crisis in institutionalised psychiatric wards, generally entails moments of crisis, more or less unexpected tensions and management problems with some group members. This makes work in co-therapy very important, and almost indispensable in the acute units, with more than two therapists if this facilitates the involvement of the nursing personnel and the better functioning of the group therapy and also of the unit (Sandison, 1994). In general, a therapy group of psychotic patients can be well directed with one therapist and one co-therapist, and professionals in training can also be accepted as observers and 'scripts'. The latter, as they progress, can act as co-therapists prior to heading their own groups. Co-therapy facilitates better observation and knowledge of the details of the group dynamics and management of transferences and contra-transferences, and also helps to solve some institutional practical aspects related with the necessary continuity of the groups due to vacations or absences.

The therapist and co-therapist should act with pragmatism and realism when they propose the creation of a therapy group with psychotic patients to the rest of the professionals of the institution. It is not a panacea or magic therapy. One should not create unrealistic expectations concerning the more difficult and resistant cases that are not going to be solved. The group cannot undertake the entire treatment of the patients included in it, and the group should not be a place where other professionals refer those patients who they not want. It is one more therapeutic resource, which has demonstrated efficacy, whose singularity and characteristics, essentially group-centric, and different from the other psychotherapies, can favourably affect the experiences and behaviour of patients with psychotic disorders (see González de Chávez, 2009; Kanas, 1996; Urlić, 2012).

When a therapy group is going to be created for persons with psychotic experiences, the therapist needs to obtain the support of the institution and to favourably motivate the centre to accept the group within its programmes and activities. The most adequate type of patients seen in this institution must be defined for the therapeutic tasks and objects proposed in the group (O'Brien, 1975). All of the group organisation needs to be explained: group strategies and techniques, referral procedure, patient evaluation and screening, the wards or offices that will be used, and the days and times available. Data should be explained regarding the most recommendable number of members, session frequency and duration, if the group is opened or closed, homogeneous or heterogeneous, if patients with other non-psychotic disorders are included, if they are hospitalised or outpatients (or if both possibilities are included), the estimated average duration of the group therapy for the group members, and how it is coordinated, in general and administratively, with the other professionals who are responsible for these patients.

It would be desirable to establish regular institutional meetings where the group therapists and the other professionals of the centre exchange information. The meetings should be adequate to coordinate pharmacological treatment and combined therapies the patient receives, whether individual, familial or socialising. These meetings should also allow the different therapists and nursing staff who participate in the patient's treatment or therapy programme to monitor the incidences, progresses or setbacks that may occur.

## Patient selection and preparation

When it comes to dealing with psychotic patients, we could be tempted to wonder, in general, when and who would recommend group psychotherapy for them (Toseland and Siporin, 1986). The specific screening of patients for a psychotherapy group is oriented so that it differentiates between the enrolment of acute hospital inpatients in the groups and the screening for outpatient groups.

In acute institutions, not all psychotic patients fulfil the conditions to participate in a group. During the most intense moments of the psychotic crisis, patients may be very disorganised, perplexed, anxious, excited, or hostile, and experience significant distortion of the context surrounding them. There is a pre-group phase of individual treatment and neuroleptic help, until the patient is capable of having a certain degree of control and better perception of the reality experienced. There is also a pre-group phase to motivate the patient to attend the group and listen to the others, in order to know that other inpatients in the centre have some experiences that are similar to theirs. This desingularisation of the psychotic experiences of the patients is the main benefit of these groups and we should facilitate it to the greatest number possible of patients, although in reduced groups, preferably having a group size of about 6 to 8 members. Initially, more flexibility with them must be allowed, because they may find it hard to remain attentive during the entire session, or it may be necessary to have greater control of their behaviour, listening to others or their interventions with the help of the co-therapists. Afterwards, these patients could disclose their experiences and compare them with those of the others, even locating them in their own biography and problems. They will have the opportunity to speak about them with other persons who have similar difficulties. They will live the experience of a group therapy context that motivates them to continue group therapy as an outpatient.

In the outpatient groups of psychotic patients, a more refined selection of the possible new members who can be incorporated into a group should be made, preferably having no more than 8 to 12 patients. In the first place, this selection will depend on the group type. This will differ, for example, for a psychoeducative, cognitive–behavioural group, or one of social activities, than for a group experiencing long-term psychodynamic orientation. The therapist who leads each group should evaluate the new candidate and his/her compatibility with the group. Additionally, the therapist should consider the rhythm when the group is opened and the appropriate time to introduce a new member in accordance with the group cohesion and process.

Although the ideal situation is that the patient enters the group after the first episode, when discharged from having been institutionalised in a psychiatric ward, and also that the same therapist or co-therapists who leads the group provides the individual treatment, since they already extensively know the patient, these circumstances do not occur in most of the institutions. Generally, other professionals are in charge of the treatment of those patients who are referred or recommended for group therapy, following written or oral protocols or procedures.

At this point, it needs to be stressed that a fluid and sincere collaboration is needed for the benefit of the patient between the professional who takes the responsibility of the drug treatment or individual psychotherapy, or the one who refers the patient to the group therapy, and the group therapist (Rand, 1999; Rutan and Alonso, 1982). First of all, it is necessary to respect the group therapist: the patient should not be sent to group therapy with concealed objectives, such as requesting a second opinion, avoiding responsibilities or simply transferring the patient. False expectations or over- or under-evaluating any of the therapies that the patient receives should not be created. Separation between both treatments (for example, considering one basic or primary and the other an accessory, sophisticated or dispensable) should always be avoided. Furthermore, a very different therapeutic relationship with both professionals, or an unshared confidentiality, should not be accepted. Even less acceptable, of course, is that the therapists communicate through the patient or the patient's family. All professionals should offer a common image of the combined therapy to the patient and family members or close relatives, in regards to both the drug treatment and the psychotherapies that the patient receives.

Prior to enrolling a new patient in the group and in addition to the information that the professional in charge can offer the patient, the group therapists or co-therapists need to have sufficient knowledge about the patient through personal interviews. They should know their psychotic experiences and biographic dynamics as well as their willingness and motivation to follow a group therapy. Lack of motivation for the group therapy by these patients should not be the initial reason to exclude them (Brabender, 2002). Instead, it is recommended that the group therapist strongly insists, both to the patient and their family members, that this unique opportunity offers benefits from being able to listen to, learn about and speak with other persons who have similar experiences. They can be given the opportunity to attend several group sessions prior to making a firm commitment. In any case, although therapeutic 'contracts' with these patients is not the norm, the therapist should ask for agreement with rules on attendance, punctuality, confidentiality, mutual respect and general group rules, which will be repeated each time another new member enters the group.

In the pre-group interviews for new group members, the usual diagnostic criteria can be discarded because they are irrelevant and do not provide the group therapist with greater knowledge about the patient or his/her possible adaptation and relationship with other group members. However, many other characteristics of the patients are important to know, in addition to their motivations for group therapy and treatment in general. For example: their degree of insight; therapeutic relationships; capacity of self-observation; psychological mentality; recovery style; personality variables; premorbid and postmorbid adjustment; social, affective, educational and occupational level and functioning; any stress and pre-cipitating factors; forms of onset and course of their psychotic experiences; and existing familial dynamics. All these characteristics are truly relevant to anticipate the future progress of the patient in the group (see González de Chávez, García Cabeza and Fraile, 1999; González de Chávez and Capilla, 2012).

The interviews of the patients with the group therapists prior to entering the group are very important to motivate and know the new members, to establish initial therapeutic relationships, to support them in their first group sessions, and to take an approach to the group therapy dynamics and processes after the patient's incorporation into the group. However, it is also important to explain the objectives of the entire therapy programme that will be followed, the meaning and details of each specific activity, and the coordination and availability of the professionals involved in all the treatment. Agreements need to be reached with the patients and family members. The group psychotherapy that they are going to initiate can be a very important therapy tool, but it is never an isolated device, so that it needs to be coordinated with all the other necessary resources for recovery.

## References

Battegay, R. (1971) 'Clinical group psychotherapy' (pp. 31–40) in *Psychodynamic Approach to Group-therapy and to Psychotherapy of Psychotics.* Copenhagen: Munksgaard.

Brabender, V. (2002) *Introduction to Group Therapy.* New York: Wiley.

Brown, D. (1991) 'Assessment and selection for groups' (pp. 55–72) in J. Roberts and M. Pines (Eds), *The Practice of Group Analysis.* London: Routledge.

Dies, R. (1994) 'Therapist variables in group psychotherapy research' (pp. 114–154) in A. Fuhriman and G.M. Burlingame (Eds), *Handbook of Group Psychotherapy.* New York: Wiley.

González de Chávez, M. (2009) 'Group psychotherapy and schizophrenia' in Y.O. Alanen, M. González de Chávez, A-L.S. Silver and B. Martindale (Eds), *Psychotherapeutic Approaches to Schizophrenic Psychoses: Past, present and future.* London: Routledge.

González de Chávez, M. and Capilla, T. (2012) 'Autoconocimiento y reacciones especulares en psicoterapia de grupo con pacientes esquizofrénicos' ['Insight and mirroring in group psychotherapy with schizophrenic patients] (pp. 125–158) in M. González de Chávez (Ed), *25 Años de Psicoterapia de Grupo en las Psicosis* [*25 Years of Group Psychotherapy of Psychosis*]. Madrid: Fundación para la Investigación y Tratamiento de la Esquizofrenia y otras Psicosis.

González de Chávez, M., García Cabeza, I. and Fraile, J.C. (1999) Dos tipos de grupos psicoterapéuticos de pacientes esquizofrénicos: hospitalizados y ambulatorios [Two types of psychotherapeutic groups of schizophrenic patients: Inpatient and outpatient]. *Revista de la Asociación Española de Neuropsiquiatría,* 72, 573–586.

Kanas, N. (1996) *Group Therapy for Schizophrenic Patients.* Washington: American Psychiatric Press.

O'Brien, C.P. (1975) Group therapy for schizophrenia: A practical approach. *Schizophrenia Bulletin,* 13, 119–130.

Rand, E.H. (1999) 'Guidelines to maximize the process of collaborative care' (pp. 353–381) in M.B. Riba and R. Balon (Eds), *Psychopharmacology and Psychotherapy: A collaborative approach.* Washington: American Psychiatric Press.

Rutan, S. and Alonso, A. (1982) Group therapy, individual therapy, or both? *International Journal of Group Psychotherapy,* 32(3), 267–282.

Sandison, R. (1994) Working with schizophrenics individually and in groups: Understanding the psychotic process. *Group Analysis,* 27, 393–406.

Toseland, R.W. and Siporin, M. (1986) When to recommend group treatment: A review of the clinical and the research literature. *International Journal of Group Psychotherapy,* 36(2), 171–201.

Urlić, I. (1999) 'The therapist role in the group treatment of psychotic patients and outpatients. A Foulkesian perspective' (pp. 148–180) in V.L. Schermer and M. Pines (Eds), *Group Psychotherapy of the Psychoses.* London: Jessica Kingsley.

Urlić, I. (2012) 'Group psychotherapy for patients with psychosis: A psychodynamic (group analytical) approach' (pp. 547–569) in J.L. Kleinberg (Ed), *The Wiley-Blackwell Handbook of Group Psychotherapy.* New York: Wiley.

Yalom, I.D. (1966) A study of group therapy dropouts. *Archives of General Psychiatry,* 14, 393–414.

Yalom, I.D. (1983) *Inpatient Group Psychotherapy.* New York: Basic Books.

# Part II

# Groups for psychoses
Different approaches and different settings

# Chapter 5

# How group psychotherapy works for people suffering from psychosis

*Manuel González de Chávez*

The distinctiveness of group therapy with persons undergoing or who have undergone psychotic experiences is the multiplicity of realities that exist in a group. There is one experience that the entire group participates in and then there are as many psychotic and unique realities as there are members of the group. How does a group like this, with such a diverse mosaic of multiple individual realities that are not shared by the others, work? How are the therapeutic objectives achieved?

## The group; an objective reality

First of all, we will say that a group is not exclusively a matrix of many intersubjectivities. It is also simultaneously and in parallell the result of many interobjective perceptions that make the group *per se* an objective reality.

The group exists in an institution. The patient has come to this centre on his/her own initiative or that of his/her close relatives, with difficulties or problems that have been evaluated by qualified professionals who have recommended that the patient attend group therapy within a therapeutic programme. The entire process – the centre, the professionals, consultations, admissions, evaluations and prescriptions – are verifiable objective facts. It is only in certain situations of crisis that the inpatients perceive this reality differently. They may perceive that the centre is not a hospital, but a jail, the healthcare professionals are disguised police, the other patients are actors, the patient has been pursued and kidnapped to kill him/her, a picture is being filmed because the subject is going to be accused, punished and shamed due to his/her behaviour or because the subject will be a relevant, admired and famous character, etc. However, with the exception of some patients and in some crisis situations, most of them consider that the roadway that has led them to group therapy is a sequence of objective events.

Group therapists and other members who attend the group are also objective realities. They have their name, professions, occupations and ages. They are men or women, are single, married, separated or divorced, they have or do not have children. They dress, have a haristyle, speak, make gestures and move in a certain way. The patients come alone or are accompanied to the consultation. They may have been inpatients, and generally take medications prescribed by specific physicians. They attend the institution on a regular basis and supposedly due to mental problems. They are in the same group room. They are real persons.

They are real persons who, according to the therapists, have similar mental problems, who can be able to understand, to cope with or to overcome these problems through the communications they establish in the group therapy. These are communications or group relations that will be institutionalised interpersonal relationships, and that will no longer be objective realities, but subjective ones. Or better stated: intersubjective ones.

## Intersubjective and interobjective communication of the group

The array of intersubjective interactions in the therapy takes place in the real world, in the objective reality (Burger, 2010). No abstract and isolated intersubjectivity exists, and the group context facilitates institutionalised interpersonal relations that are intersubjective and interobjective, aspects that, as in any human relationship and in any therapeutic relationship, function in a joint, parallell and mutually dependent way (Buirski and Haglund, 2001).

All the group members, including the therapists, are real persons. Even though a patient, at a given moment, may have a distorted interpretation of them, this does not mean that they are no longer the persons they really are, with their objective and verifiable data and characteristics. That said, everything they communicate about themselves as observations and reflections on their life and experiences or those of other group members are no longer so objective and verifiable, but rather are mostly subjective perceptions that may or may not be intersubjectively validated.

Supposing, as it should be, that the group does not consider its members as mere dysfunctional brains or as carriers of artificial nosological entities, but rather as persons with problems and biographical difficulties, what they describe will never be objective truths because, with the exception of some data or dates, no objective biographic truth exists. The biographic experiences of others, in general, and that of the group we are now discussing, cannot be verified through interpersonal communication. We can only know about them, recognise them and perhaps validate them by consensus. The group dynamics and process will never be a sequence of objective truths, but rather it is the product of the intersubjective communications of the real persons who make up the group, the joint construction of a collective reality formed by narratives and interventions of the group members, including the therapists, whose degree of truthfulness, at first, is not sanctioned or questioned. They are admitted as subjective truths.

In a group with persons with psychotic experiences, the psychotic experiences themselves are true for those who experience them, and the other group members should accept them as such. To make this happen is one of the first tasks of the therapist, who should encourage group cohesion and acceptance among the members, creating a group culture of mutual respect, empathic listening, reciprocity, sincerity and confidentiality in the communications (Urlić, 1999). It is only in this way, within a receptive, respectful and safe context that the patients can emerge from their defensive withdrawal and usual lack of trust, and venture to disclose their psychotic experiences to the others in the group.

## Self-disclosure of the psychotic experiences

There has already been some disclosure of some psychotic experiences by the patient before he/she enters the group. These may have been verbally disclosed, or manifested through their behaviour to their relatives: a perception or interpretation so different from reality that it finally gave rise to a professional consultation. In other cases, a public incident has been the cause for psychiatric commitment. Afterwards, now within the institution, and in a group of specific interviews, some disclosures of the patient have led to diagnosis and therapeutic recommendations, which include group therapy. Furthermore, and before the patient enters the group, the therapists have been able to know, at least partially, the psychotic reality that the patient lives or has lived. This is, for the patient, an objective reality, although neither the patient's relatives nor the healthcare professionals see it or believe it to be true. Nonetheless, in this entire pre-group stage, the person with psychotic experiences has already been considering whether he/she should reveal them or not. The patient has been questioning if this will provide any relief or help, if by doing so the truth of his/her experience could be verified, or if this would only entail diagnoses, stigmas, rejections and disqualifications. That is why it is common for these persons to have an attitude of uncertainty, suspicion and fear of incomprehension when they enter the group.

Group therapy facilitates self-disclosure for the patients (Vinogradov and Yalom, 1990). The patients are going to have the opportunity to listen to other biographical accounts and the psychotic experiences that the other group members have lived or are living within a climate of mutual respect. The group horizontality and reciprocity make it an active, multifocal and multi-intersubjective context that is very productive in identifications among its members and associations derived from their narratives and disclosures. The participant can observe his/her own similarities and differences, but above all, it is possible to observe how others listen closely to the unique experiences of others, and all the reflections and respectful questioning with which they try to know, understand and give credibility to these supposedly objective truths or realities that are the psychotic experiences of each person.

As in other therapies, self-disclosure by the patients greatly depends on their personal dynamics, defensive self-control and risks they believe are involved, or their will and expectations of clarifying and verifying their experiences. However, it also depends on the attitude, empathy, interest and commitment of the therapists (see Derlega and Berg, 1987; Farber, 2006) and of the other group members. Self-disclosure of the patients is not linear, but rather it is a spiral personal process, which will gradually emerge during many sessions. Generally, the patient first communicates those aspects that cause him/her more stress or are less painful, and then later exposes his/her fragility and the traumas to which shame and guilt is attached. Nonetheless, we should not indulge in the simplicity of making elementary correlations between the self-disclosure in the group and the prognosis of the psychotic patients (Donald, et al., 1975). The prognosis of the patients is the result of many personal and care variables. Self-disclosure, which regulates and protects privacy and identity, is an intersubjective variable that moves within the parameters of the advantages and risks of each interpersonal relationship and each context. It is an interpersonal process, and in this case, a group one, which greatly depends on the recipients or confidants. It also depends on the attitude of listening, attention, discretion, trust and empathy of the other group members.

## Insight on the others

The self-disclosures of the patients concerning their problems and biographic and psychotic experiences facilitate group cohesion as well as other therapeutic factors, such as catharsis, universality, identifications or interpersonal learning (Bloch and Crouch, 1985). All this gives rise to *mirroring*, probably the most specific phenomena of group therapy (see Pines, 1982; Berger, 2012), which is the intersubjective and interobjective process of multiple simultaneous and reciprocal mirror reactions between the group members, who listen, observe, explore and are getting to know each other.

What makes the multiple dyadic, voluntary and intended relationships within the group generate the mirror phenomena is that the group members share the same or similar disorders or difficulties and that they live or have lived some similar experiences. This means that each patient can be a mirror for the others, and the other group members can be mirrors for the patient, who sees in them some of his/her own problems, reactions and behaviours, as well as the perceptions and interpretations that the patient shares with the others and other particular experiences that are not shared in any way. Mirroring facilitates observation and examination of similarities and differences within the group: that which is in common with others or with all, that which only happens to some of its members, that which is experienced in the same way, or that which is experienced differently. It simultaneously facilitates knowledge of others and knowledge about oneself, and forcibly obligates the person to think about the others and to think about oneself.

As each group member discloses his/her psychotic experiences within a climate of listening and respect, it soon becomes clear that some perceptions or interpretations of the reality cannot be accepted by the others as true verifiable objectives. For example, supposed powers to move the stars, to make it rain at will, to provide love and happiness to all humanity, and to end wars, poverty or unemployment. Other psychotic disclosures such as the voices they hear, or the telepathic influences or power they cause, experience or suffer, are also not validated by consensus in the group. Those who are living these experiences initially attempt to convince the others of their reality. Those who do not experience them try to understand them, examine their origins and characteristics, and compare them with other contrary evidences or other possible interpretations.

In response to the non-acceptance by the others of the reality of their psychotic experiences, some patients will try to encompass all the group in their delusion, which the group will rapidly reject by showing other evidence. Others will try to confirm and reinforce the psychotic experiences of other members in order to have their own experiences accepted as real. The interventions of the therapists should contrast and disassemble this rhetoric of psychotic reinforcement, for lacking data and credibility. The reinforced patient will often participate because he/she picks up on a hasty fallacy of the person trying to validate what he/she barely knows.

The mirroring in a group of psychotic patients exploits the possibility of *insight*. A patient can quickly and very easily recognise the psychotic experiences of the others but at the same time is incapable of recognising his/her own psychotic experiences. The patient can separate the duality of the external and internal world in the others, as well as their desires and fears of the facts: the objective reality they perceive in the others and the psychotic rhetoric with which they communicate and cannot verify. This is a duality, an objective and subjective reality, in which each patient cannot distinguish in themselves those aspects of their experiences and identity in which their own reality has been subjectively transformed (González de Chávez and Capilla, 2012).

## Acceptance of the subjective character of the psychotic experiences

Perhaps initially, with some surprise and confusion, each group member sees that he/she cannot ratify the truthfulness of the psychotic experiences of the others and also observes, through the insight of the others, how the rest of the group questions the veracity of his/her own experiences. The experiences described by group members may have many similarities, and they also have one thing in common: no one can verify the unique world that the others live and so all believe the psychotic experiences of the others are unreal.

Group dynamics, full of unique worlds that cannot be collectively objectified or validated by consensus, creates a combination of multiple perplexities for the group and an increase of the internal contradictions of its members. Some will doubt themselves, others will insist on their psychotic convictions, and others will want to devaluate the opinions or experiences of the others. The therapists should lead the group from the questioning of the reality to consensus of the subjectivity, to the accepting of the subjective character of the psychotic experiences. These personal and unique experiences are realities truly lived by each one. They are subjective realities. The acceptance of the subjective character of the psychotic experiences is the first, essential and inexcusable objective of group psychotherapy with persons who suffer psychotic disorders. In the group, each patient begins to question his/her own uniqueness when questioning the unique world that the others experience. They begin to doubt the objective reality of their psychotic experiences when doubting the objective reality of the psychoses of the others.

Accepting the subjective character of the psychotic experiences opens a new world of questions to the group and to each of its members. How and why have they arrived to this subjective transformation of their own realities. How and why a particular member of the group, and they themselves, experience some specific aspects of reality in a completely different way to the others. It is the group and personal process travelling from the psychotic identity and reality, with a lack of insight, to the contradictory internal debate on the reality or unreality of the experiences, that leads to the acceptance of the subjectivity of the disorders.

The group now begins to question the causes of the disorders *per se*. It is no longer a reflection on the veracity, but rather on the causality. It becomes an internal reflection of each one on themselves, their identity and life, and a common reflection, thanks to the interpersonal learning in the group on biographical dynamics, internal conflicts, vulnerability factors and precipitating circumstances that have led them to the crisis. The group therapy becomes a personal and group process of self-observation and self-knowledge (Garcia Cabeza and González de Chávez, 2009).

## From the vulnerable identity to the integration of the identity

The process of self-observation and self-knowledge in the group is always an unequal process because the psychotic experiences are heterogeneous and the capacities and characteristics of each one of the group members are unequal. There are patients who cannot, or resist, exploring deeper the factors that have influenced their disorders. Others are initially inclined towards general or non-specific physical causes, such as stress, tiredness or insomnia, and others still persist in magical causalities, such as voodoo or the evil eye, or openly psychotic ones, such as intentional poisonings. All can accept that they have been or are vulnerable and, based on this recognition, the therapists should work to homogenise the group as much as possible, but to avoid disturbing the rhythms and processes of each member too much.

In the dynamic oriented groups, the group process is focused on interpersonal, familial and social psychological factors existing in each of the members. The self-disclosures are now more biographical related, with the fragilities and adversities lived, and with the coping strategies and mechanisms used most to defend identity and self-esteem. Multi-intersubjective and multifocal group therapy is very productive and considerably accelerates the opportunities of reflection and self-knowledge. However, these processes are not easy for the psychotic patients who have often used strategies of negation and self-deception when faced with their problems and conflicts in their lives. In the psychotherapy programmes, only a minority achieve an understanding of the sense and meaning of their psychotic experiences (Alanen, et al., 1986): that is, to integrate them as part of their new identity, and to connect these experiences as the uncontrollable manifestation of the rejected, denied, regressive or idealised aspects of themselves that forced the psychotic collapse of their vulnerable identity.

Nonetheless, most of the psychotic patients in a group therapy are able to achieve a less vulnerable and more autonomous, realistic and stable identity. They are less likely to seek unreal subjective solutions and more capable of coping with their difficulties with realism. They are more opened to and capable of introducing those changes into their lives and their relationships that facilitate their recovery. This is because the objective of the group psychotherapy is not only the collective reflection that leads to self-knowledge, but also the common reflection that leads to action.

## References

Alanen, Y.O., Räkkölainen, V., Laakso, J., Rasimus, R. and Kaljonen, A. (1986) *Towards Need-Specific Treatment of Schizophrenic Psychoses.* Heidelberg: Springer Verlag.

Berger, M. (2012) 'The dynamics of mirror reactions and their impact on analytic groups' (pp. 197–216) in J.L. Kleinberg (Ed), *The Wiley-Blackwell Handbook of Group Psychotherapy.* New York: Wiley.

Bloch, S. and Crouch, E. (1985) *Therapeutic Factors in Group Psychotherapy.* Oxford: Oxford University Press.

Buirski, P. and Haglund, P. (2001) *Making Sense Together: The interpersonal approach to psychotherapy.* New York: Jason Aronson.

Burger, T. (2010) *Origins of Objectivity.* Oxford: Oxford University Press.

Derlega, V. and Berg, J. (1987) *Self-Disclosure: Theory, research and therapy.* New York: Plenun Press.

Donald, S., Strassberg, M.A., Roback, H.B., Anchor, K.N. and Abramowitz, S.I. (1975) Self-disclosure in group therapy with schizophrenics. *Archives of General Psychiatry,* 32, 1259–1261.

Farber, B. (2006) *Self-Disclosure in Psychotherapy.* New York: Guilford Press.

Garcia Cabeza, I. and González de Chávez, M. (2009) Therapeutic factors and insight in group therapy for outpatients diagnosed with schizophrenia. *Psychosis,* 1(2), 134–144.

González de Chávez, M. and Capilla, T. (2012) 'Autoconocimiento y reacciones especulares en psicoterapia de grupo con pacientes esquizofrénicos' ['Insight and mirroring in group psychotherapy with schizophrenic patients] (pp. 125–158) in M. González de Chávez (Ed), *25 Años de Psicoterapia de Grupo en las Psicosis [25 Years of Group Psychotherapy of Psychosis].* Madrid: Fundación para la Investigación y Tratamiento de la Esquizofrenia y otras Psicosis.

Pines, M. (1982) Reflection on mirroring. *Group Analysis,* 15, 1–26.

Urlić, I. (1999) 'The therapist role in the group treatment of psychotic patients and outpatients: A Foulkesian perspective' (pp. 148–180) in V.L. Schermer and M. Pines (Eds), *Group Psychotherapy of the Psychoses.* London: Jessica Kingsley.

Vinogradov, S. and Yalom, I. (1990) 'Self-disclosure in group psychotherapy' (pp. 191–204) in G. Stricker and M. Fisher (Eds), *Self-Disclosure in the Therapeutic Relationship.* New York: Plenun Press.

# Chapter 6

# Transference and countertransference features in a psychological approach to patients with psychosis

## The group-dynamic considerations

*Maurizio Peciccia, Ivan Urlić, Simone Donnari*

## Introduction

According to the results of much research, generally speaking the most positive outcomes for patients with psychosis can be obtained by combining medication and psychotherapy. The psychotherapeutic approaches can be dynamic/non-dynamic, supportive, psychoeducational, or other types of rehabilitation. It is important to underscore that the psychodynamic approach stems from the psycho-analytic concept of understanding the developmental line of a human being, from prenatal observable phenomena and following all life phases. Primarily, this includes object relations theory, ego- and self-psychology, and attachment theory, among others. The understanding of the developing human being and the crucial importance of the constant interaction between its genetic endowment and the surrounding enviroment represents the inexhaustible source for observation and analysis of multiple influential elements that in different developmental phases shape one's personality traits, relational patterns and behaviour, as well as that of groups.

Clinical and neuroscientific research has shown that the human brain stores all impulses, favourable and unfavourable, and that is not able to 'forget' anything, if not organically damaged. Freud believed that forgotten is not lost, because it is preserved in the unconscious. This means that all experiences shape human understandings and reactions that are in constant active intertwining, either on the conscious or unconscious level, when understanding oneself and/or relating to the environment. These features Freud recognised as mental mechanisms that manifest themselves as transference and countertransference phenomena, which together with defense mechanisms, the structural model of personality, function-ing of the self, the psychological features of groups, type of object relations and attachment styles, represent the basis of psychodynamic approach. Foulkes, as psychoanalyst, describes the group as an important and valuable therapeutic tool, applying psychoanalytic concepts, and adding some group-specific phenomena, such as group-as-a-whole, group matrix and group resistances, as well as specific therapeutic factors, and transference and countertransference features in the group setting. Although group analysis was created for patients suffering from neurotic disturbances, through time its applicablity has included other patients with 'difficult diagnoses' like patients suffering from borderline and psychotic disturbances.

## On transference and countertransference of patients with psychoses

Since Freud introduced the notion of transference in 1912, many important authors have described different facets of the phenomenon. Fenichel (1945) writes that transference unfolds inside and outside analysis, in persons with neurosis, psychosis, or in healthy people. All human relationships contain a mixture of realistic and transference reactions, like the primitive, archaic and essential derivatives of the early relationship mother–child. Many or even all elements of an object relation could be contained in a transferential relationship. Basically, the transferential reactions are repetition of object relations from previous times. An expression of the possibility to re-experience repressed and frustrated instincts and inhibitions, it represents expression, rather than the avoidance of recollection, defence from remembering, and manifestation of repetition compulsion (Freud, 1912, 1914; Freud, 1937; Fenichel, 1945). Greenson (1967) wrote that transference is an anachronism, a mistake in time. It is pertaining to the transfer, impulses, defences and emotions connected with a person from the past toward a person from the present, and that the phenomenon is unconscious.

Psychic processes that are intertwined in the transference have some constant features: repetition compulsion, the object on which the emotions are transferred, projection with transferred emotions, transference situation and regression. The characteristics of the transference are its inadequacy, intensity, ambivalence, instability and persistence. It is important to bear in mind that repetition always represents a resistance toward the function of recollection. Followers of the Kleinian school see transferential phenomena like projections and inprojections of very immature objects of good and bad quality. The patients showing this kind of transference are not communicating with a coherent, integrated ego, and do not seek to establish a working alliance but the direct contact with various introjects. Searles (1965) writes that transference includes three persons: the subject, the object from the past, and the present object. In essence, the matrix of transferential relationships is the primal union of mother–child.

The transferential phenomena are based on two elements: the capacity of differentiation between self and the world of objects, and the capacity to transfer emotional reactions from object representations from the past to the present object. The transference relationship to the therapist, though regressive and ambivalent, represents the essential factor for the establishment and continuation of treatment (in this respect, the initial contact with the therapist can play a decisive role through the perception of introjected 'good' or 'bad' characteristics) (Urlić, 1999, 2016). The more that the transference is regressive, the more space will be occupied by aggressive instincts. Benedetti (1991) writes that psychotic transference means not only a repetition of the past, but also the real relationship which conceals the new beginning.

Transference can be positive or negative. Due to the deficit in the ego function, the patient uses primitive mechanisms of defense like negation, massive projection, projective identification, splitting and primitive idealisation. This means that there is no possibility of integrating 'all good' and 'all bad' representations of self and object in integral representations, so that object constancy cannot be reached: thus, integrated objects are experienced as partial (Žunter-Nagy and Mayer, 2001). The object relationships can be of 'motherly', 'fatherly', 'brotherly', etc., quality. The transferential reactions could be distinguished according to the phase of the development of libido, or regarding the structure: the analyst/group conductor could become representative of superego, of ego, or of identification, for the patient or the group. The identification should also be included in transferential reactions.

---

## Distinguishing identification in the field of psychosis

*Clinical vignette 6.1: Psychotic transference*
The psychotic transference occurred when the newly admitted patient, due to exacerbation of his psychosis, joined the therapeutic community group on the ward spontaneously. He insisted on participating in the session. All of a sudden he jumped off his chair, trying to throw it in the direction of the team of therapists, screaming to the psychiatrist that he is the head man who has insulted him this morning. The chair broke the window glass, which stirred fear in the group, until the very agitated patient was taken out of the room.

*Clinical vignette 6.2: Transferential psychosis*
The patient was sent back from the army because he was 'not suitable' for army service. His weird behaviour was showing unfavourable progress. In an outpatient group of patients suffering from psychosis, he declared that he had decided to discontinue the group. When asked for an explanation, he declined to say it in public. The therapist suggested that he should write down his reasons for the next session. At the next session, very reluctantly, the patient, supported by the therapist, started to read from his paper, often stuttering and blushing: 'doctor, you are the worst person I have ever met, the dirtiest character, the most untrustful person . . .', and all of a sudden he switched his tone to: 'doctor, you are the nicest person I have ever met, the most trustful friend, my father, my brother . . .'

---

In the group setting, there are some special phenomena of expressing transference, for example: multiple transferences, transference to the group-as-a-whole, transference of the whole group, pairing, subgrouping, alternative sessions, dreams and silence. As regards transferential resistance, features include: the 'requirement' for transferential gratification, the defensive transferential reactions, generalised transferential reactions, acting-out of transferential reaction (as in Case vignette 6.1), and acting-out in the analytic situation (ego-syntonic) (as in Case vignette 6.2).

As a rule, the transference should be analysed when it: represents resistance, attains an optimal level of intensity, or when the psychotherapist's/group conductor's intervention will add a new insight. For the patients with psychosis, the technique of intervention needs to wait until the patient/group is mature enough to bear confrontation with the use of arguments. It should be underscored that the 'unsolvable' transferential reactions occur in cases of error in the evaluation of the capacity for transference, in erotic transference or in masked perversion leading to psychosis (Štrkalj-Ivezić and Urlić, 2015).

The elaboration of the negative psychotic transference is often a time of crucial importance, not only for the first phase of therapeutic process, but for the whole course of the therapeutic relationship and cooperation. In this context, we ascribe particular meaning and importance to establishing: a 'corrective symbiotic experience' (Urlić, 1999, 2012; Štrkalj-Ivezić and Urlić, 2015); the regulation of proximity and distance; and reliability, nonintrusive attitude, empathy, and other characteristic features of the psychodynamic processes in the therapeutic relationship. The symbiotic transference is kept out of consciousness because it can activate intolerable feelings of fragmentation and therefore persecutory defences. The dual transference of the psychotic patient, both fusional–symbiotic and autistic–separative should also be analysed (Peciccia and Benedetti, 1996). Fusional transference/countertransference is often viewed as a defence against separation that evokes the ghosts of annihilation and death fears. When, on the other hand, the therapist/therapeutic team is dominated by autistic transference/ countertransference, characterised by disinvestment of the others and by feelings of worthlessness and helplessness, it is possible to grasp behind these manifest features levels of fusional–symbiotic elements which are split off.

Countertransference is a key issue for the therapist/therapeutic team, who cannot remain 'untouched' by many highly specific and deeply regressive symptoms of different pathological features of patients with psychosis. These features often trigger very intense, even stormy, feelings that can cause confusion in the therapist/therapeutic team, and difficulties in controlling them. The role of the therapist/therapeutic team requires acceptance of some specific attitudes (Urlić, 1999, 2012). It is important that (group) psychotherapists learn how to recognise, elaborate and make constructive use of what they have understood from their reactions and feelings. The containing capacity of the therapist/therapeutic team, especially in relation to group psychotherapy with psychotic patients and groups for family members, needs continuous supervision and opportunities for consultation (peer-supervision).

Gabbard and Wilkinson (2000), underscore that the successful approach and management of countertransference in the treatment of difficult patients depends primarily on holding (Winnicott, 1945) and containment (Bion, 1962). The contemporary notion of holding in its very essence bears a movement from the concrete to the symbolic. For that development to occur, Bion's description of how the mother processes the affects of her infant holds key importance as a result of the need for the mother to help the infant to avoid unmanageable pain. Bion believed that when the mother returns unmodified affects to her infant, the infant is likely to feel persecuted by the return of the projected contents, and may experience fragmentation of the self as a result.

The patient in the situation 'here and now' unfolds his early experiences and wishes to intertwine the therapist, which in him/her stimulates different intensive feelings – a countertransferential reaction. To contain the highly ambivalent and fast-changing transference, to be the container that detoxifies patient's negative and dangering contents, to endure patient's non-neutralised aggression, to accept the regressive fusion and repetitive establishment of boundaries, to adjust to oscillations in patient's functioning during developmental phases, to preserve psychotherapeutic function when often endangered by the patient's behaviour – all this (according to Žunter Nagy and Mayer, 2001) requires great psychic efforts from the therapist. As a result, the therapist/therapeutic team must protect him/themselves, and supervision, peer consultations and self-analysis are of the utmost importance.

In the psychopharmacological era, medication, besides its biochemical value and place in a comprehensive therapeutic approach, has important emotional meanings and should also be considered in relation to transitional phenomena (in the Winnicottian sense).

## The thrapeutic context

In various group therapeutic contexts, it is possible to create protected spaces, initially external to the patient, where his/her split-off fragments of the self may be placed, in order to dream them and sew them up in the relationship with the group or the therapist/therapeutic team. The setting varies according to the degree of the patient's fragmentation. If speech is not compromised, it is possible to use verbal psychoanalytic group psychotherapy. If the patient cannot speak, but can draw, we can use group art therapy. Sometimes, when the patient can neither speak nor draw, we use a new form of communication: amniotic therapy.

### Amniotic therapy

This is a group therapy that takes place four times a week in water heated to 35°C (Peciccia and Benedetti, 2006; Peciccia and Donnari, 2006; Donnari, Garis and Peciccia, 2006). Amniotic therapy may reactivate memories of contact with amniotic fluid and with the uterus. The group becomes a symbolic uterus which contains and supports. Amniotic therapy offers the patient physical and mental holding which was not interiorised during childhood. Amniotic holding is based upon repeated movements of union and separation. In the beginning, the fluctuations between union and separation in water can be perceived sometimes as anguishing and frightening, and sometimes as safe and protective. The patients, held by amniotic operators, are united, separated and then again re-united with other participants. The shifts and overlapping of bodies in water generate continuous merging and separation. An amniotic therapy patient described his experience:

> Sometimes I felt like losing my consciousness and shifting in a dreamlike state, and I felt surprised to somehow wake up in the water. I was not really sure whether it was a dream, because a part of me was conscious. I could describe it this way: I didn't know anymore where I was and I had a dream because I could see dreamlike images. But while I was dreaming I was not losing my consciousness. It happened to me for three or four times in a row. And I felt faithful of not drowning.

This patient's experience underscores the importance of the basic trust and feeling of security between the patient and the therapist. Immersed between being awake and asleep, every patient and the entire group experiences a concrete, physical form of dream-work (see Chapter 10). Amniotic therapy activates dream-work, in pairs and in a group, and helps patients to interiorise (to contain and integrate) a constant loving presence of others that supports and contains.

Evidence-based assessments of amniotic therapy showed a global increase in patients' quality of life and social skills (Peciccia, et al., 2015). Improvement in social skills in the group of amniotic therapy participants seems related to the improved ability in defining *self-boundaries*. Two factors trigger self-boundaries enhancement. The first, nonspecific, is the presence of water acting like amniotic fluid that can give containment and protection. The second trigger is a peculiar way of body holding that pertains to the method. There are two kind of amniotic holding: individual and group. The patient can be held and hugged either by an operator, or by more than one group participant, or else by the whole group. Amniotic holding is never just symbiotic: in the hug, next to merging contacts skin-to-skin, there are always movements of micro- and macro-separation. A patient described self-boundaries:

> This way of being gently touched is very unique. It somehow defines me on a sensorial dimension; it works like a body map, actually my body map. I mean it is the external boundary of my own body and the fear of feeling my own body, which is both a landmark and a map that I'm discovering. This sort of learning how to feel myself gives me the impression of discovering parts of myself that I never experienced before and maybe this really works, and if so, it is far beyond the intellect. It is something that has nothing to do with the intellect.

Amniotic holding triggers strong parent–child transference and countertransference movements, thanks to a six time reduction of body weight due to submergence in water. Memories related to holding a baby or being held as a baby are stimulated. When patients are ready to verbalise, they are encouraged to undertake a psychodynamic psychotherapy in a group or individually.

---

### Clinical vignette 6.3: Paternal transference in amniotic therapy

Patient G is 25 years old. In his early childhood, he was taken away from his violent and dangerous father, but continued to live with his mother. He is afraid that the father might come back, and that it could come out of the blue. When this thought becomes stronger, he even loses blood in his urine. G is not able to socially connect; he is frightened of being in a group of people. Every attempt of social integration has failed because when he is surrounded by people, a sort of mental scene arises: a horror film where he is the victim. After amniotic therapy, G states:

> It was a very special experience; a type of body experience that I can define as 'paternal'. The kind of physical experience that a person can experience being held by his father. For example, it was as if I was with my father this morning after I do not even know how many years, and it was truly a gift. I could describe it with just one word: balance. A strong feeling of balance that I haven't felt for a long time and it's like having another body.

*Comment:* The amniotic therapy group offered containment for his horrifying projections and transformed them to love and protection. For the first time, G feels to be in the right place for releasing his nightmares, to dream them and to digest them with the group.

In a complex experience, G is then capable of being supportive towards the therapist, who feels like a sister in need of protection. In a countertransference, the therapist feels like G is a brother, capable of protecting her, and associates the emotional experience with her painful childhood (when she felt anything but protected by her older brother, who in reality had sexually abused her for years). In this case, more than transference and countertransference took place: it was a reciprocal transference. The supervision was therefore crucial in deepening the understanding of these experiences.

---

In amniotic therapy, we have also observed an activation of the sublimation of erotic instincts both in patients and in therapists. In the sublimation, the aim of the genital instinct is displaced and, both in patients and in therapists, the genital pleasure transforms itself into the pleasure of being held, cradled, the feeling of skin when it is touched by the warm liquid, and by the whole group's amniotic containment. The desexualised energy produced by sublimation follows various paths:

- In the therapist, it increases the devotion towards the patient, who is supported and held with more care and affection. In this case, the sublimation energy of the genital instincts is put into the service of feeding the patient's pregenital needs.
- In the patient, the desexualised energy produced by the sublimation of the genital instincts is addressed towards the therapist holding the patient.
- The desexualised energy produced by the sublimation of the genital instincts is also directed towards the group and can be observed in the increasing of contacts among group's participants and in the rhythm and the frequency of the unions–separations within the group. Thus, the sublimated energy of the genital instinct is put into the service of the primary process of repairing in the group. A fragmented and threatening container turns itself into a whole maternal body, in a holding-with-love womb.

### Art therapy

In conclusion, we will present some images and comments from Patient C, who has shown through art therapy his experiences during amniotic therapy. These meaningful images can help to understand the emotional intensity of this work, and the emotions that can be triggered both in the patient and in the therapists.

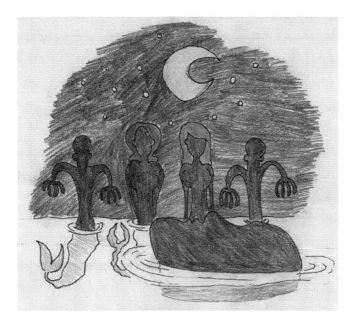

*Figure 6.1* 'This is the pool under the starry sky and represents the feeling that I had while I was with my eyes closed: that mermaids were around me ... The figures here are black because you could not see their faces, and they may be either friendly or threatening as you can see from the position of the hands. The faces instead were merely like emerging masks.'

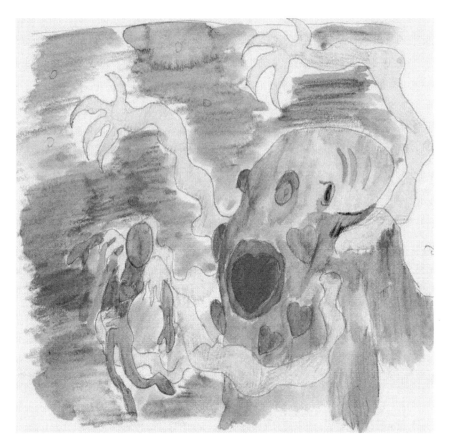

*Figure 6.2* 'Underwater, the noise of the heartbeat is always amplified and the feeling of the group comes from all these hearts beating as one. It seems somehow the sound of a creature which you see in my drawing. It is not a monster but a good one, giving massages to people with seaweed hands. So the hands are delicate rather than monstrous. The creature has several hearts beating.'

The 'bad thoughts', fears and threats that are now being projected in the group take a tentacular form. Yet the creature also has delicate arms, 'like seaweed', and, most importantly, the beating hearts signify the start of some emotional closeness in the group. The warm support is symbolised by the red heart of the patient, which is also drawn on the the monstrous figure.

The warmth of the water is the sign, and not the symbol, of affective warmth and of the heart of the group. Emotional closeness begins to be experienced as pleasant and not threatening. This group experience allows the patients to live symbiosis and separation at the same time, integrating them together.

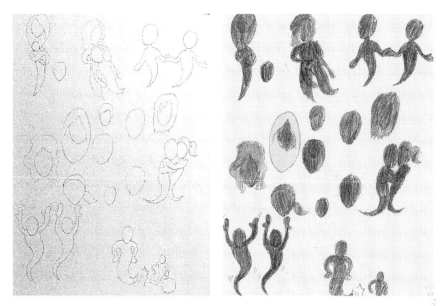

*Figure 6.3* 'This drawing has a deeper meaning. It represents various sensations of the therapy. There are many faces that symbolise the community, the possibility of getting together and feeling as one. There are some hugs between the mother with the child, two friends, a mother and an older son, a boyfriend and a girlfriend and, a person with a child playing – who could be me with my grandson. The contact and the hug in the water suggests to me other situations where this occurs.'

In this image, a sequence of many transference moments experienced in the group are represented: infant–son, brother–friend, son–teenager, but also a lover and father. The 'bubble' containing the group seems to be strong, and opens the doors to positive experiences. In group therapy in the water, these transference positions are embodied by men and women who share an experience of relationship with the patient's pain, with his death and life. During the therapeutic work, it is the therapist's ability to integrate these functions that allows the maintenance of a deep alliance with the vital psychic resources of the patient, often hidden in his symptoms.

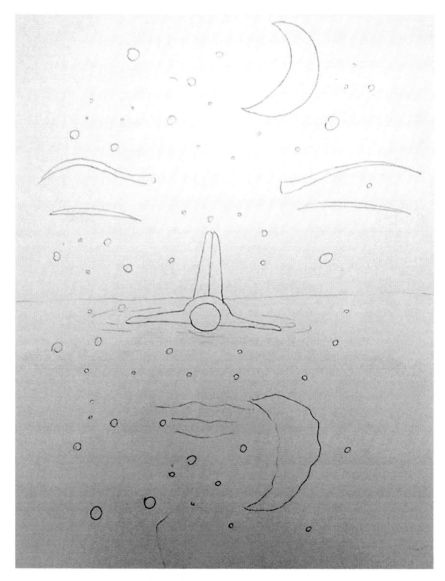

*Figure 6.4* 'This drawing works on three levels. There is a man floating on the water with his legs raised. There is also the night sky reflection on the water. Altogether it also represents a sleepy face. There are the eyes, signs in the water for the mouth and the man is the nose. Everything has a dreamlike dimension.'

In this last image, a face emerges from an intricate web of group identifications and counter-identifications. The image recalls the well-known saying: 'the whole is more than the sum of its parts'. It seems to represent Foulkes' opinion (in reference to Lewin's studies on the concept of field, dated to the 1930s), that the originality of the group situation does not depend on the sum of the personalities of each member. Instead, the 'matrix' shows its own structure and functional autonomy that somehow transcends the individual, even if it is completely built and shared by the individuals. The group has a strong inner complexity, even if the group is also a functional unity.

During their complex therapeutic paths, psychotic patients encounter different professionals in various contexts of care. The fragmentation of their existential experience compels them to spread out parts of their own self and their inner world. These disconnected pieces can be considered pieces of a confused mosaic, waiting to be re-ordered to reflect the patient's identity and consistent integration. In Figure 6.4, the coming out of a unique face shows the slow process of identity construction. The verbal and non-verbal group experiences, as mentioned above, help the patient to 'dream outside', integrating experiences of symbiosis and separation. We try to re-assemble a mosaic, thus allowing the patients to identify with an unitary image of their own self that can be internalised as a safe and steady symbol (Donnari, 2011).

The care that is constantly shown towards the primordial affective needs of each patient, and for their progressive differentiation, like the evaluation of important relationships, enables the therapeutic group members to maintain a plastic and multidimensional internal representation of the patient that is always prone to further integration. It represents an extremely safe basis that enables the patient to unleash the old consolidated representations of her/himself in order to reach different ones; ones that are wealthier and more authentic.

## References

Benedetti, G. (1991) 'Foreword' in G. Benedetti and P.M. Furlan (Eds), *The Psychotherapy of Schizophrenia.* Cambridge, MA: Hogrefe & Huber Publishers.

Bion, W.R. (1962) *Learning from Experience.* London: Heinemann.

Donnari, S. (2011) 'Video-integration in group therapy of psychoses' (pp. 40–53) in *17th ISPS International Congress 'Psychological Therapies for Psychoses in the 21st Century Influencing Brain, Mind and Society'.* Dubrovnik, 31st May–4th June.

Donnari, S., Garis, M. and Peciccia, M. (2006) Warm water dipping group therapy for psychotic patients. *Acta Psychiatrica Scandinavica*, 431(114).

Fenichel, O. (1945) *The Psychoanalytic Theory of Neurosis.* New York: Norton.

Freud, A. (1937) *The Ego and the Mechanisms of Defence.* London: Hogarth Press.

Freud, S. (1912) 'The dynamics of transference' in J. Strachey (Ed), *The Standard Edition of the Complete Psychological Works of S. Freud*, Vol. XII (1978). London: Hogarth Press.

Freud, S. (1914) 'Remembering, repeating and working-through (Further recommendations on the technique of psychoanalysis II)' in J. Strachey (Ed), *The Standard Edition of the Complete Psychological Works of S. Freud*, Vol. XII (1978). London: Hogarth Press.

Gabbard, G.O. and Wilkinson, S.M. (2000) *Management of Countertransference with Borderline Patients*. Lanham, MD: Jason Aronson.

Greenson, R.R. (1967) *Technique and Practice of Psychoanalysis*. New York: International Universities Press.

Peciccia, M. and Benedetti, G. (1996) The splitting between separate and symbiotic states of the self in the psychodynamic of schizophrenia. *International Forum of Psychoanalysis*, 5, 23–38.

Peciccia, M. and Benedetti, G. (2006) Principio del piacere e psicosi [Principle of pleasure and psychosis]. *Rivista di Psicologia Analitica*, 74, 87–118.

Peciccia, M. and Donnari, S. (2006) 'Ad aquas – Le acque della salute' ['Ad aquas – The waters of health'] in *I Nuovi Luoghi delle Cure a Cura di Pier Maria Furlan* [*The New Place of Care by Pier Marian Furlan*]. Turin, Italy: Edizioni Celid.

Peciccia, M., Mazzeschi, C., Donnari, S. and Buratta, L. (2015). A sensory-motor approach for patients with a diagnosis of psychosis: Some data from an empirical investigation on amniotic therapy. *Psychosis*, 7(2), 141–151.

Searles, H.F. (1965) *Collected Papers on Schizophrenia and Related Subjects*. New York: International Universities Press.

Štrkalj-Ivezić, S. and Urlić, I. (2015) The capacity to use the group as a corrective symbiotic object in group analytic psychotherapy for patients with psychosis. *Group Analysis*, 48(3), 315–331.

Urlić, I. (1999) 'The therapist role in the group treatment of psychotic patients and outpatients. A Foulkesian perspective' (pp. 148–180) in V.L. Schermer and M. Pines (Eds), *Group Psychotherapy of the Psychoses*. London: Jessica Kingsley.

Urlić, I. (2012) 'Group psychotherapy for patients with psychosis: A psychodynamic (group analytical) approach' (pp. 547–569) in J.L. Kleinberg (Ed), *The Wiley-Blackwell Handbook of Group Psychotherapy*. New York: Wiley.

Urlić, I. (2016). 'The single session approach: The importance of the first encounter between patient and the doctor'. Lecture at the School of Psychotherapy of Psychoses, Dubrovnik, Croatia.

Winnicott, D.W. (1945) Primitive emotional development. *The International Journal of Psychoanalysis*, 26, 137.

Žunter Nagy, A.M. and Mayer, N. (2001) 'Transference and countertransference in psychotherapy of psychoses'. Lecture at the School of Psychotherapy of Psychoses, Dubrovnik, Croatia.

# Chapter 7

# Group psychotherapy in the acute inpatient unit

*Ivan Urlić*

## Introduction

In principle, psychiatric services are organised to be centred on either hospital services or on a network of mental health centres that includes an intensive connection with the hospital ward. In any case, if hospitalisation is needed to protect the patient and the surroundings from hetero- or auto-aggressivity, or some other form of uncontrolled behaviour and influence of pathological aberrations in experiencing internal or external worlds, or both, the patient suffering from acute psychotic episodes is most often confronted with the ambience of the acute psychiatric unit.

The understanding of the psychopathology of patients with psychosis and the possibility for better treatment in the acute state of decompensation involves the following considerations:

- The meaning of the hospitalisation.
- The value of the first encounter for patient–therapist/therapeutic team.
- When and how to communicate that the patient's inclusion in the therapeutic community of the acute psychiatric unit is expected.
- How to convey to the new patient that the freedom of verbal expression of one's thoughts and feelings excludes acting-out.

The first encounter(s) between the psychiatrist/psychiatric team and a patient has a great and decisive value in determining the possibility of cooperation between them, or between groups of patients with psychosis and the conductor, hospital nurses and therapeutic team.

## The first encounter for patient–therapeutic team: Individual and group experiences

Research into the working alliance in psychotherapy owes much to complex new understandings of the meaning of the emotional vulnerability of persons who can later develop dissociative and psychotic ways of coping with early traumatic experiences (González de Chávez, 2012), and to new understandings offered by neuroscientific discoveries. These experiences, with their imprinted memories and consequences, tend to surface in hypersensitive persons as symptoms that are expressions of deep dissociative and split-off mechanisms of defence. Psychotic symptoms dominate their clinical pictures.

## Clinical vignette 7.1

The patient was admitted as an emergency case accompanied by family members, medical staff and police. He was a young person, extremely agitated and expressing his enormous fears, cursing and spitting, and trying to get rid of his custodians. He was refusing any verbal contact and immediately after being fixed to the bed and receiving medication, I explained my responsibility for his admittance in the hospital and that his

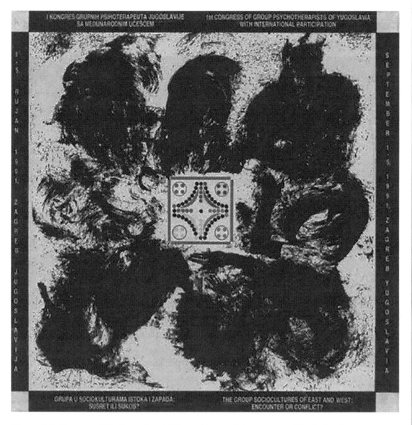

*Figure 7.1* Poster with Rorschach-like stains and the game of Ludo in the centre.

fixation was in order to prevent any harm that he could provoke on himself or others. I told him that the team would help him to calm down, and then we would talk about his experiences. Some other patients from the unit reassured the newcomer that he could be confident that this promise would be kept.

After several days, the patient was invited to talk with the psychiatrist. On entering the room, his sight was absorbed by a poster (see Figure 7.1), which was inspired by Rorschach stains. In the middle of the poster, the game of Ludo represents well-structured play. After some time, the patient said that he felt 'like this', and pointed to the turbulent part of the design. I nodded. He continued: 'and you would like me to be like this', indicating the well-structured game. I nodded again. The patient let a sigh of relief and sat down, willing to enter into a dialogue. This was the beginning of successful cooperation. Later on, during therapeutic community encounters, he was very constructive in encouraging other newcomers to be cooperative in treatment.

*(Source:* Urlić, 2012)

The working alliance is an aspect of the therapeutic relationship that deals with collaboration (Manor, 2010). In individual consultation or groupwork, such collaboration has to develop not only between the therapist and (each) patient, but also among all the patients who attend each group. Each patient is expected to receive help not only from the psychiatrist or the therapeutic team, but also from his/her peers (family members, friends, workmates, other group members, etc.).

While the first medical contact for the acutely psychotic patient is usually one-to-one, groups are also inevitably present: family, medical and social professionals, including police and emergency medical services, other patients from the psychiatric unit, etc. (Urlić, 2012). Mutual trust building is the core element in enabling individual patient or group members to disclose difficulties and to establish secure and trustful relationships with important persons in their environment. The group members should become aware of the corrective emotional experience within the therapeutic setting, individual or group, and should compare diverse kinds of experiences (even the corrective symbiotic experience) (Urlić, 1999, 2012; Štrkalj-Ivezić and Urlić, 2015).

After more than 40 years of work in the psychiatric service, the psychiatrist can recollect all sorts of encounters with different psychiatric cases. These encounters are usually of patients accompanied by family members, or police and medical emergency services where they are needed to intervene. Rarely does someone decide to consult a psychiatrist about feelings or symptoms concerning changes in thinking and other elements of cognitive sphere that are puzzling and burdening that person, sometimes even in an obsessive way.

## Clinical vignette 7.2

Sometime ago I received a phone call from a distant town. The name was not unknown to me, but I could not recollect any more details. The young male person introduced himself as an engineer, living with his family and working in that town. He had a stable marital relationship and two children of school age. He was satisfied with his job and expressed his vision for profession advancement. He was in regular contact with his psychiatrist in order to receive medication. The only dissatisfaction, he said, was about not having the opportunity to talk about his thoughts and feelings: he felt tormented all the time, with different intensity.

He was phoning me because he remembered the first encounter he had with me, 15 years ago, when he was first brought to the psychiatric clinic in psychotic decompensation with suicidal intentions. This happened during the first year of his being a student. Coming from a traditional family with four children, he had never left his village for a long period until he started his studies. This first separation from his family and living ambience stimulated in him intensive anxiety, unmotivated fears and suicidal ideations. During our first interview, his hypersensitivity could be recognised, along with separation anxiety and fears of psychotic intensity. High doses of pills controlled his suicidal ideations and attempts. After discharge from the hospital, he continued his studies in another city where he had family members and medical support.

Now, 15 years later, after having his family, job and a satisfactory life, he wanted to talk about the threat that he was feeling inside. He recollected that his father used physical punishment during his childhood and adolescence, along with frequent criticism and no praise. His low self-esteem was stimulating his suicidal impulses. Becoming aware of this connection, and through emotional elaboration, the pressure of these ideations lost their intensity and his self-respect could grow. During his psychotherapy, he repeatedly underscored that our first encounters had helped him to transform fear of psychiatric therapy into the empowering feeling of human closeness with the psychiatrist. Hence, corrective emotional experience appeared to be the essential supportive element during and after many years.

According to Satir (2000),

> The whole therapeutic process must be aimed at opening up the healing potential between the patient and the therapist/therapeutic team.

In my experience, nothing changes until that healing potential is opened: the meeting of the deepest self of the therapist with the deepest self of the patient.

This creates a context of vulnerability and of openness to the possibility of change. Moreover, Satir (2000) describes a simplified definition of a system – a kind of continous dialogue:

> . . . action, reaction and interaction, amongst a set of essential variables that develop an order and a sequence for a joint outcome.

Agreeing with a tendency toward positive eclecticism, Kanas (1996) advocates an integrative approach that would include all the constructive elements from all the types of approaches in the group psychotherapy of patients with psychosis. The strengthening of ego functions by means of group therapy, especially the possibility of feeling and testing reality, still remains the basic aim of this approach. In other words, coping with symptoms and improving interpersonal relationships should be constantly worked upon as basic aims of treatment. In this way, psychopharmacotherapy and psychotherapy represent two parts of a whole, together with psychosocial interventions.

---

## Clinical vignette 7.3

More than 30 years ago I encountered an architect who, even as a student, was prominent among his colleagues. His career proceeded in a brilliant way. He lived with his family, and was father to three children. His psychotic crisis surprised his family, but was not a suprise to himself. Over a period of many years, he was sometimes aware that he was not able to fully function. Rather grandiose fantasies had a disorganising effect on his work and creativity. He was very worried that he could not contain these episodes, and was anxious that his wife, children, friends and collaborators would perceive his 'absentmindedness'. In actual fact, his affectivity was rather flattened and he was perceived as an introverted person. At the begining of our therapeutic cooperation, he accepted that he was not 'free' in his behaviour and in expressing his feelings and ideas due to dissociative symptoms that were making him different from people around him.

After several years of psychotherapy combined with small doses of antipsychotic medication, we agreed that he would attend consultations only when he felt in need. After many years, he reported to me that he was regular with his very reduced medication, and that in diverse moments he spoke to me in his imagination, as if he was in our psychotherapy experience. During all these years, he had become a very renowned architect and was functioning very well. The favourable impressions from our first encounters had de-dramatised his thinking about the psychotic side of his mind, so that he was able to live and work with small amounts of psychiatric help.

The structured, albeit regressive, hospital environment represents a framework for the symbiotic experience, which in the corrective and constructive sense offers the following (Urlić, 1999; Restek-Petrović, Orešković-Krezler and Mihanović, 2007; Gans and Counselman, 2010):

- A structured, personal and dyadic relationship with the doctor and medical personnel (if adequately trained).
- Medications, which in addition to their pharmacological effects are also imbued with the meaning of a transitional object that is often ambivalently invested and incorporated. Consequently, medication can be experienced independently of their pharmacological properties.
- The group experience, as a place of exposure, as well as the possibility of 'practising' a triadic situation, which determines the assessment of the patient's capacity for social re-adjustment, or the defusion level of partial objects and the degree of establishing their integrity and constancy.

Most frequently, hospital treatment also represents a selective element for the continuation of group psychotherapy in outpatient treatment.

## The relationship between a patient with psychosis and the therapist

In the application of individual or group psychotherapy to patients with psychosis, the following are of fundamental importance:

- The assessment of the patient's capacity to establish a relationship with the therapist and, through him/her, also with others.
- The personality traits and training of the therapist.

The capacity of a patient with psychosis to establish a relationship with another person primarily refers to the capacity for introjection. The integrity of a patient's intrapsychic experience is interwoven with his/her capacity to perceive the outer reality and to introject the therapist from this reality as a separate external object. Another dimension of the relationship to the outer reality is projection, which is interwoven with introjection. The constant exchange of introjection and projection determines the experience of the self and the definition of external objects and the environment. According to Satir (2000):

> You affect and you have an effect.

The capacity to establish relationships with others is related to the possibility for patients suffering from psychosis to establish positive transference (see also Chapter 6). Transference of the patient with psychosis will also include repetition of the relationship to the therapist/therapeutic team from their first encounter(s), with elements from real life (see Clinical vignette 7.2).

The therapist should introduce the following therapeutic features into the therapeutic relationship (Urlić, 1999, 2012):

- Unpossessive warmth (in a primary, unidirectional and nonverbal capacity).
- Empathy (the therapist's capacity to introject the patient as an object and to structure the image of the patient with as much data as possible from all developmental phases: the image of the patient in the therapist is shaped through the arrangement of nonverbal and verbal data perceived unconsciously and consciously).
- A genuine aspect (enabling the therapist to direct and measure his/her behaviour toward the patient spontaneously).

Conducting a group of patients with schizophrenia or some other psychosis, the therapist acts differently than in a group of persons able to function at a higher level. The aims of group work are related to the specific needs of the patients. Due to the difficulties patients with psychosis have in experiencing and interpreting both inner and outer realities, Kanas (1996) describes the functions of the therapist in such groups. The therapist is: (1) active and directive in keeping group members focused on the topic; (2) clear, consistent and concrete with interventions; (3) supportive and diplomatic with comments; (4) open and willing to give opinions and advice that are appropriate to the discussion; (5) here-and-now (rather than there-and-then) focused; and (6) encouraging of patient-to-patient (rather that patient-to-therapist) interactions.

Within the context of the therapist's role in a group of patients with psychosis, there is a dilemma between the two basic types of conductor: 'energiser' and 'provider' (Yalom and Lieberman, 1971). In terms of measured action, it seems that the patience of the provider is more acceptable (Urlić, 1999), as it appears that the therapist's role as a 'new primary object' is more adequately realised in this way, although it requires fuller and longer engagement from the therapist.

In consideration of small- and medium-sized groups of inpatients and outpatients suffering from psychosis, as well as the therapist's role in such groups, the following could be said (Urlić, 1999, 2012):

- The therapist conducts the individuals in the group. From experience, this situation does not change considerably from the beginning to the end of group treatment under hospital conditions, due to the deep regression and fragmentation of the psychic functioning of the patients. In an outpatient group, a more flexible approach is possible, with the transformation of the open ended into a more defined course of treatment.
- In hospital groups, due to time constraints in terms of ward treatment and heterogeneity in the regression depth, the therapeutic aims are necessarily limited. In constrast, an outpatient group needs constancy or spatial and

temporal continuity, with an open and adjustable perspective at the level of ego functions and stability in the patient's object relations. In an outpatient group of patients with psychosis, the possibility for the evolution of the therapist's role from leader to conductor is more realistic and often more adequate than under hospital conditions (Foulkes, 1964). This means that the distinctions between these two types of conduct become more amenable to a wide range of influences and, therefore, considerably more flexible in their exchange.

• Therapeutic work in a group setting can be aimed at corrective symbiotic experience, as well as at the 'dilution' of the dyadic transference relationship in terms of development directed at a triadic, better socially adjusted level (Urlić, 1999; Chazan, 2001; Štrkalj-Ivezić and Urlić, 2015).

• Under both hospital and outpatient conditions, group psychotherapy of patients with psychosis, together with psychopharmacological therapy, represents an essential complementary part of the treatment of patients with psychosis (with the exceptions of manic patients or those inclined to acting-out, and with questionable benefits to patients suffering from acute paranoia). The social component of the biopsychosocial approach should always represent one of the basic working frameworks, having in mind the best possible level of recovery.

• Group psychotherapy of patients suffering from psychosis represents an important part of both the diagnostic and therapeutic procedures. It can represent a technique for a professional approach as part of the usual routine or it can reach high levels of creativity and represent a challenge for further scientific research.

Therefore, the psychodynamic (group-analytic) approach should be considered to be the body of concepts stemming from essential psychoanalytic notions and a wealth of long-term clinical experiences, subject to appropriate modifications when the psychodynamically oriented group psychotherapy of patients with psychosis is in question. According to my experience, this is the most efficient way of supporting social functioning and personal identity, leading to recovery.

## Clinical vignette 7.4

In an inpatient group psychotherapy session for patients with psychosis, Patient L relates her dream. She is going to a party. Many of her friends will be there. She is curious to see who she will encounter. In the next scene, she is meeting her friend (who suffers from schizophrenia and has attempted suicide several times) who greets her: 'Hello, how are you?' In this dream, he is very normal; a man of culture and very intelligent.

After having related her dream, Patient L adds that she is still puzzled and excited that a 'crazy' person can feel so well and appear so normal. In the group discussion, many patients agree that they sometimes feel normal and sick at the same time. This is a sign of hope for each of them. The therapist then emphasises the importance of continous cooperation with the therapeutic team. Many group members nod.

After a brief silence, Patient M says that she would like to share her secret: she was divorced because she couldn't bear to live with a rigid man. She has had many partners since then. Her mother, a widow, says that women should not be alone. Comments in the group concern difficulties in establishing more stable relationships within their families. Sometimes these difficulties result in the avoidance of close interpersonal contacts. Another group member proclaims that he feels good in this group due to his confidence in all the team members and the group.

*Comment:* In this session, mutual trust building was the core element in enabling group members to disclose their difficulties in establishing secure and trustful relationships with important persons in their environment. The group members were becoming aware of the corrective emotional experience within the therapeutic group and could compare diverse kinds of experiences.

(*Source:* Urlić, 2012)

## Goals, tasks and bonds for psychotherapy inpatients with psychosis

The inpatient framework leads the therapist to constantly ask how the various systems involved (the patients, the therapist, ward staff, families, patients' employers, etc.) influence and, in turn are also influenced by, three major issues: goals of group work (psychotherapy), tasks (i.e., the methods) chosen, and bonds that develop during the session (Manor, 2010). The atmosphere of the psychiatric unit as the therapeutic community creates an important impact on the nature of relationships and the whole setting, leading to the working alliance. Warmth when approaching patients should be communicated constantly, verbally and non-verbally. Due to rapid turnover of patients, the atmosphere may fluctuate from one moment to the next, requiring new adjustments. This reflects on the group as a whole, influencing goals, tasks and bonds.

Due to the specific characteristics of the nature of work on the acute psychiatric unit, goals have to be modest as regards the expectations of patients, and what can be achieved during their hospitalisation. Problem-solving skills are an important part of the group work, aiming to strenghten patients' ego functions and reality testing. MacKenzie (1997) suggests that tasks can be planned in a 'single session format', where each session is a self-contained experience. It should be kept in mind that inclusion of the newly admitted patient too early might provoke in him/ her new fears and projections, and projective identifications, which might result in acting-out behaviour that could be not only disruptive for the group, but also even dangerous due to released aggressivity.

Group work in the acute psychiatric unit reflects mostly some previous experiences of each member of the group. It is important to use group work as a privledged place in which to support the making of new acquaintances and to experience the possibilities of social bonding. The holding and containing function of the group, as well as of the whole unit, and the structuring function of boundaries and working alliance are usually helpful in this respect. In this environment, the reduction of splitting and deeply regressed personality function-ing is encouraged, so that patients can re-establish better reality testing and the capacity to inter-relate with other people. Although this starts in the well struc-tured and protected therapeutic experience in the acute psychiatric unit, it can later function in recognisable group culture.

## Concluding remarks

Considering the group characteristic of human nature, patients with acute psy-chotic decompensation on an acute inpatient psychiatric unit, should be met by a well structured acceptance of their unthinkable fears, anxiety and feeling that his/her life is endangered. The patient's structured therapeutic acceptance should include:

*   Clearly defined treatment modalities.
*   Medication, and a system of neutralisation for possible or explicit auto- or hetero-aggressivity.
*   Appropriate explanation, on an individual basis, of the working alliance that is proposed by the unit.
*   Group experience, in order to foster bonding with other patients and the therapeutic team, as well as to re-establish or support the capacity for social re-adjustment.

The containing capacity of the unit should consider boundaries and the unit's structure, as well as the precarious balance between hierarchy and democratic elements, especially with patients who are in acute psychotic decompensation or otherwise functioning with a blurred sense of boundaries. Special attention should be given to those patients who respond with refusal towards the warm acceptance, which can indicate that the patient is overwhelmed with paranoid fears. To regulate distance in relationship with paranoid and very agitated patients is part of routine work in an acute inpatient psychiatric unit. This is especially important when group work is in question.

All group work in an inpatient psychiatric unit takes place in situations that are constantly changing. The main goals of this group work with psychotic patients can be listed as to:

- help patients to overcome acute psychotic crisis;
- enable patients to re-establish better equilibrium in psychic functioning;
- ameliorate reality testing;
- better regulate affects' modulation and behaviour patterns;
- improve interpersonal bonding;
- prepare patients to continue with group psychotherapy as outpatients;
- strenghten ego functions and social connectedness.

The creation of a positive experience from the (first) encounter with the acute psychiatric unit is a challenge that includes constant support for the shift from excessive use of primitive towards more mature mechanisms of defense. The classic group-analytic approach should always be adapted to take into account the specific needs of patients diagnosed with psychosis (either of schizophrenia, bipolar or some other etiological source).

## References

Chazan, R. (2001) *The Group as Therapist.* London: Jessica Kingsley.

Foulkes, S.H. (1964) *Therapeutic Group Analysis.* London: George Allen & Unwin Ltd.

Gans, J.S. and Counselman, E.F. (2010) Patient selection for psychodynamic group psychotherapy: Practical and dynamic considerations. *International Journal of Group Psychotherapy,* 60(2), 197–220.

González de Chávez, M. (2012) '¿Cómo establecer relaciones terapéuticas con una persona que vive experiencias psicóticas¿' ['How to establish therapeutic relationships with a person who experiences psychotic episodes?'] (pp. 361–381) in M. González de Chávez (Ed), *25 Años de Psicoterapia de Grupo en las Psicosis* [*25 Years of Group Psychotherapy of Psychosis*]. Madrid: Fundación para la Investigación y Tratamiento de la Esquizofrenia y otras Psicosis.

Kanas, N. (1996) *Group Therapy for Schizophrenic Patients.* Washington, D.C.: American Psychiatric Press.

MacKenzie, K.R. (1997) *Time-Managed Group Psychotherapy.* London: American Psychiatric Press.

Manor, O. (2010) 'The single session format' in J. Radcliffe, K. Hajek, J. Carson and O. Manor (Eds), *Psychological Groupwork with Acute Psychiatric Inpatients.* London: Whiting and Birch.

Restek-Petrović, B., Oreškovic-Krezler, N. and Mihanović, M. (2007) Patient selection for group psychotherapy of patients with psychosis (Croatian). *Socijalna psihijatrija,* 35(3), 133–139.

Satir, V. (2000) 'The personhood of therapist: Effect on systems' in B.J. Brothers (Ed), *The Personhood of the Therapist.* Philadelphia: Haworth Press.

Štrkalj-Ivezić, S. and Urlić, I. (2015) The capacity to use the group as a corrective symbiotic object in group analytic psychotherapy for patients with psychosis. *Group Analysis,* 48(3):315–331.

Urlić, I. (1999)' The therapist role in the group treatment of psychotic patients and outpatients. A Foulkesian perspective' (pp. 148–180) in V.L. Schermer and M. Pines (Eds), *Group Psychotherapy of the Psychoses.* London: Jessica Kingsley.

Urlić, I. (2012) 'Group psychotherapy for patients with psychosis: A psychodynamic (group analytical) approach' (pp. 547–569) in J.L. Kleinberg (Ed), *The Wiley-Blackwell Handbook of Group Psychotherapy.* New York: Wiley.

Yalom, I.D. and Lieberman, M. (1971) A study of encounter group casualties. *Archives of General Psychiatry,* 25(1), 16–30.

# Chapter 8

# Short- and long-term group psychotherapy for outpatients suffering from psychosis

*Marjeta Blinc Pesek, Bojana Avguštin Avčin,*
*Nada Perovšek Šolinc, Kaja Medved*

## Introduction

Group psychotherapy for outpatients with psychosis has proven to be beneficial for the patients and is rewarding for the therapists. It can be applied in different settings and can have different short- and long-term goals. The duration of group psychotherapy, as well as inclusion and exclusion criteria, and therapeutic technique and goals, are all important considerations when planning to work with a group of patients with psychosis. We report on our experiences and findings with intermediate and long-term groups of outpatients suffering from psychosis.

## Selection of patients

Patients rarely seek group psychotherapy on their own initiative. Sometimes a family member, usually a parent, searches for the 'best' treatment for their 'ill' child, but it is mostly the therapist who selects the patients, based on those individuals who he thinks could benefit from group work. An important factor for successful and rewarding group therapy of patients suffering from psychosis is that the group member is treated in regular psychiatric care, which includes individually prescribed medication. A positive prognostic factor is regular communication between the treating psychiatrist and group leader.

In the initial, preparation phase for the group, each candidate for group therapy should have at least one or two individual preparatory sessions. If the group is led in co-therapy, both co-therapists should be present. The therapists should be familiar with the patient's detailed psychiatric history as well as social and living conditions. It is important to motivate the patient and asses the level of ego functioning and reality testing, as well as the intrinsic motivation for group therapy. The patients with psychosis suitable for short- and long-term group psychotherapy form a heterogeneous group, as regards to their level of social functioning, phase of psychotic process, personality features, hospitalisation experiences and other life circumstances.

The goals for each group vary, but they all have a common purpose: to increase patients' awareness of themselves through interaction with other group members who provide feedback on multiple levels – responsiveness, engagement, emotional control or spontaneity – and on their behaviour in general. Through group interactions, patients improve their interpersonal social skills. The feelings of stigma and isolation decrease. All this can improve the patients' quality of life. Long-term groups can promote changes to the deeper levels of psychological structure of patients, and improve their basic trust.

It is known however, that not all patients with psychosis can benefit from group psychotherapy. Among relative contraindications are severe paranoid symptoms, acute psychotic illness, deeply depressed, impulsive borderline and narcissistically structured patients, as well as those who are psycho-organically damaged. For patients with these disturbances, homogenous groups are indicated according to the diagnosis; while for patients with other psychotic features, heterogeneous groups of male and female patients are recommended (Urlić, 2010). Exclusion criteria for outpatient group psychotherapy are substance-abuse comorbidity, severe comorbid dissocial personality disorder, need for chronic hospitalisation for symptom control, significant cognitive impairment or organic mental syndrome.

## Setting

The recommended size of group is 6 to 8 members, but in practice it varies from 3 to 12 members. Frequency of sessions varies from weekly to fortnightly meetings. The duration of the weekly groups is 60 minutes and the fortnightly groups meet for 90 minutes. Groups may be open or closed as regards the inclusion of new members. Intermediate-term groups are usually closed groups. The setting and goal should be made explicit in the preparatory sessions and repeated in the first group session. Long-term groups are usually slow open groups, meaning that a new member can be included after a previous members' termination. The setting and goals should be reviewed at the beginning of every new members' first session (see Bernard, et al., 2008).

## The therapist

The group therapist working with patients with psychosis should be genuinely interested in, and empathetic with, the patients and the group. However, he should be capable of maintaining the appropriate level of distance (Gabbard, 2005; Štrkalj-Ivezić and Urlić, 2015). Patience to wait for the very small and slowly coming changes that patients achieve is essential. It is important that the therapist can contain the strong affects and projections that patients suffering with psychosis often express in group therapy.

The therapist should be trained in group psychotherapy, especially when working with long-term groups where elements of group analysis emerge and deeper insight is sometimes achieved by members. It is important to have some experience with treatment of patients with psychotic disorders and to undergo regular supervision. Therapists should be: (1) active in keeping group members focused on the topic; (2) clear, consistent and concrete with interventions; (3) supportive and diplomatic with comments; (4) open and willing to give opinions and advice, as needed and appropriate to the discussion; (5) here-and-now focused; and (6) encouraging of patient-to-patient interactions.

There are some benefits to conducting groups in co-therapy. The co-therapeutic pair is usually formed of a therapist experienced in conducting psychotherapeutic groups for patients with psychosis, and a co-therapist or assistant, who can be less experienced. The co-therapeutic pair should function as a good team, working through any potential conflicts between themselves. In co-therapy, it is easier to deal with and contain the strong affects and unconscious and unspoken conflicts that often arise in groups and are unbearable for the patients. The therapist pair can maintain reality inspection and ensure continuity, which is very important in the treatment of patients with psychotic disorders.

There are some important modifications to the group-analytic technique that are used when working with patients suffering from psychosis. We practice a modified, non-structured, psychoanalytic group technique with components of psychoeducation, cognitive elements, non-structured conversation, and clarifications and encouragement of interactions between group members. Only a few group interpretations are made, and dynamic interpretations are avoided even if the therapeutic relationship is strong. The therapist is active, offering more educative interventions and clarifications, and even some direct suggestions and gratifications can be helpful (see Kanas, 1996).

---

### Clinical vignette 8.1

Patient A, a 35-year-old female with schizophrenia, became a member of the therapy group during her mother's terminal illness. She took over all the care and responsibility for her mother during her illness. At the time of her mother's death, she received support in the group. Patient A moved back to her own apartment after her mother's death and started to work.

PATIENT A: I was tortured during my hospitalisation on the secure ward.
THERAPISTS AND REST OF THE GROUP (*trying to explain the situation*): You were delusional.
PATIENT A (*got upset*): It was terrible. They were torturing me; it was horror.
PATIENT A (*to the therapist*): I demand that you believe me!
THERAPIST (*reassuring, with calm voice*): Yes, I believe you.

*Comment:* Patient A was attempting to project her distress and fragment-ation, still in denial of her mother's loss, to the therapist. The despair that she felt when she was psychotic and hospitalised 5 years ago, and her mother could not prevent it or relieve her pain, is repeated now in her psychotic transference toward the therapist. The content of her despair, which was the loss of her mother, had yet to form. She demanded her pain to be recognised and contained. This was achieved by not interpreting her delusional belief of being tortured.

Interactions among group members are actively encouraged. The focus should stay on the here-and-now themes that are important for the members. The therapist should try to include all members of the group in discussion, assisting the silent members to speak, as well as to understand the reasons for their silence. When the members interact spontaneously around an appropriate issue, the therapist should stay silent and allow the patients to feel a sense of mastery and independence. When there is conflict between members, the therapist should not take sides but rather encourage the whole group to discuss the issue in a way that leads them to understand why the conflict has arisen. The therapist's task is to help the group develop into a cohesive unit with an atmosphere where curative factors can operate. In this way, the group becomes the therapist (Urlić, 2010; Yalom and Leszcz, 2005).

## Short- and intermediate-term groups

Intermediate-term groups are defined as groups that run from 10 to 12 months; all groups that are planned for a shorter period of time are called short-term groups. New patients are usually not introduced during such a short period, but some flexibility is appropriate. Short-term groups integrate well with individual psycho-therapy, cognitive training, family support and other psychosocial interventions used in the treatment of early stages of psychosis.

Short-term psychotherapeutic groups are often designed as skill-training groups. An example is the FETZ (The Cologne Early Recognition and Intervention Center for mental crises) programme (Addington, Francey and Morrison, 2006), where groups are run as skills-training groups as part of an outpatient inter-vention programme for the treatment of the early prodromal stages of psychosis. These groups offer the members peer models for dealing with stress, symptoms and perceived stigma. For many members, it is very important that group therapy offers the opportunity to experience that they are not alone in their illness and problems. Working through feelings of stigma due to mental illness is an important group task.

The conceptual framework for short-term group work is based on the vulnerability and stress-coping concept of schizophrenia. Cognitive-behavioural interventions and metacognitive training strategies can be used in short-term groups. The specific aim of groups in the very early stages of psychosis is to improve symptoms, to prevent social decline and to prevent or delay progression to acute psychosis. Hence, improving coping resources and stress management are underlying strategies of the intervention. Patients recovering from first-episode psychosis can also benefit from short-term group interventions. In these cases, the aims of short-term groups are to help patients develop social skills, to offer education about the illness, to develop an understanding of the impact of the illness on their lives and to re-evaluate their goals and ambitions. It is important for patients who have experienced psychosis to have the opportunity to share their experience with others.

The educative elements that are often used in the first stages of group therapy help patients to cope with their psychotic symptoms. Topics related to treatment, medication, their traumatic experiences or their specific needs are discussed in a safe environment. Other, especially optimistic, everyday topics are encouraged. The group members improve their communication skills; they learn to listen and develop better reality control. They interact in a group environment where a regression-preventing structure is provided through the interventions of the therapists.

We use our modification of the integrative model of group therapy (Kanas, 1996, 1999), which is supportive in nature. Our groups can be run as intermediate-term groups of 8 to 12 months in duration. In the first phases of psychosis, patients gain better control and differentiation of their psychotic symptoms and emotions, and improve their social functioning (Addington, Francey and Morrison, 2006). Group cohesiveness develops very slowly, but once formed it remains very strong (Lakeman, 2006). A very important feature of intermediate-term groups is that they relieve the enormous distress and suffering of patients with psychosis, especially in the first and intermediate stages of the disease. In these stages, many patients mourn their loss of health, aspirations and ambitions that they held before the illness developed.

On an interpersonal level, it is important to help the members to become less isolated and to improve their relationships through the group interactions. Healing comes through the experiences that the patients have with each other during the sessions, and through immediate feedback from the therapists in the here-and-now context. The sessions improve group interactions in everyday life, which improves social functioning. By developing a more 'normal' communication style, and better and more stable relationships, the members reduce self-stigmatisation and improve self-awareness and ego functioning.

The integrative model of group therapy uses open discussion, where members choose and develop the topics themselves. Long-term problems and maladaptive behaviours may be examined. It is important to use psychodynamic understanding of the individual patient's history, as well as for the ongoing dynamics in the group.

## Clinical vignette 8.2

A small, intermediate-term group of patients with psychosis was held in the psychiatric clinic Rudnik, Ljubljana, for 8 months. The group was run in co-therapy. The co-therapeutic pair consisted of an experienced psychiatrist and a psychologist. A modified, non-structured, psychoanalytic technique with free-floating discussion, psychoeducation and clarifications was used. After two drop-outs and one premature termination, three constant male members formed a firm group matrix. All of the included patients were diagnosed as having schizophrenia or schizoaffective disorder based on DSM-IV diagnosis criteria.

During the first four sessions, the main topic was psychosis – its causes, consequences and the fear of it. Members talked about hospitalisations, their psychotic episodes and medication: *I felt stigmatised after I had been hospitalised and tied up three times.* In the next sessions, members shared their feelings of trauma that could not be expressed in their previous social context. They vocalised being misunderstood, feeling lonely, and their guilt about putting their families in the position of stigma and shame: *After my psychotic episode, I isolated myself. I thought that no one could understand what had happened to me and I did not want to cause trouble for my family.*

At the tenth session, members agreed that it was not easy for them to come to therapy. They were all anxious because it was hard for them to freely express their negative feelings. They recognised their impulse to withdraw from the group and from the discussion: *It's easier not to come to the group, or to come and be quiet: but this is not why we are here.* A similar topic occurred at the twelfth session, when one of the members expressed his feelings about his thoughts: *Sometimes I am ashamed of my own thoughts. I wish to be invisible when that happens.*

*Comment:* We were able to observe the member's affective desire to be 'unseen', as well as a perception of being deeply flawed and incapable. The member functioned on the neurotic level at that time, and expressed feelings of shame, but this situation had no important influence on the group process or on the discussion, because other members were not at the neurotic level.

After analysing the group process and focusing on shame, we wanted to point out that we were able to recognise three phases in the group process: (1) the first phase concerned psychosis – its causes, consequences and the fear of it; (2) the second phase concerned stigma – the members vocalised both feelings of loss for their social role and status, and trauma connected to their psychotic episode; and (3) the last phase concerned differentiation – a potential to work with personal themes connected to shame. One of the members expressed some thoughts of which he was ashamed, but at that time, he was the only group member in full remission (functioning on a neurotic level); and therefore we were unable to work on shame at a group level. Another important factor to note is the length of the group therapy. This group lasted 8 months, a period of time that is not long enough to address personal themes connected to feelings of shame. Yet despite this, members were able to verbalise feelings of guilt for putting their families in the position of stigma and shame.

In this kind of group, we can work on stigma, feelings of loss and trauma. Members can differentiate their psychotic content. They can also differentiate their position in the group and in life. This leaves the patients with opportunities to choose a long-term group and to continue working on the psychotherapeutic process.

The time limit of the group can accelerate the group process, and in the termination phase we could observe grandiosity and feelings of excessive love among group members, in contrast to their feelings of distrust towards the outer world. Their 'healthy parts' communicated about their need for love and connectedness. Taking into account that groups function on the level of its weakest member, it was an important conclusion for us that the personal themes of shame could not be resolved unless all the group members are in full remission. In this group of patients with psychosis, shame was present at an unconscious level that could not be reached and addressed.

## Long-term groups

Long-term groups are carried out for many years; some last for even more than a decade. Long-term group work has important short- and long-term effects on quality of life, compliance with treatment, social functioning and stigma reduction (Martindale, et al., 2002). Patients should be intrinsically motivated and well prepared for group work (Lakeman, 2006). Long-term groups can evolve from the patients who participated in short- or intermediate-term groups and can be slow in progression and open ended. New members are included after a previous member has terminated the group.

With the progression of group process, we observe more constant membership, and honest and open conversation about symptoms and real-life problems. Some patients may leave the groups early, but the remaining members are constant and some of them may feel unable to end the group process. After termination, the patients may engage in social networks that continue some of the beneficial effects of the groups. However, some patients develop transient worsening of their psychotic symptoms during group therapy.

We have clinically observed the best outcome for patients who attend these groups for 3 to 5 years. Some patients who stay in groups for more than 6 years may be unable to separate from the group and move on to social settings outside the group. Our clinical observation is that the patients who stay in the group for longer than 6 years had less social interaction outside the group or immediate family. There may be an optimum time at which the patient should leave the group, depending on the level of functioning in the group and outside the group (Blinc Pesek, et al., 2010). For patients for whom the group represents the only social interaction outside the immediate family, day care centres or clubs may be an alternative.

In our experience, we have found that these groups are more important to the more severely ill patients, which indicates that the recovered patients do not rely on group therapy as much as the patients with some degree of illness or disability. Patients in long-term groups get to know each other well; trust and cohesiveness develop over time. Since long-term group therapy helps patients to develop better insight into their illness and more self-awareness, they usually develop long periods of stable remission. This enables the therapist to stimulate a controlled level of regression and anxiety, which brings primitive defence mechanisms and object relations to the surface. Yet the group also functions on the free-floating discussion level, which means that we can observe the same group phenomena as in groups of patients with less severe diagnoses. The therapist will control these phenomena in order to prevent relapses.

---

## Clinical vignette 8.3

Patient U, a male 36-year-old group member, with a serious form of schizophrenia, has been absent from the group for several sessions. At the beginning of his absence, he let the group know that his absence was due to a relapse of his illness. Later on, despite being absent from the group, we did not hear from him for four sessions. The group talked about Patient U, and members expressed their concern and asked the therapists to invite him to return to the group. Several female members of the group expressed their wish to have his phone number so that they could contact him and ask him to return to the group. Eventually, it was the therapist who invited him to return to the group. The first session after his return:

PATIENT U *(turned towards the therapist)*: Something is happening to me. From your neck up I can see my mother's head.
ANOTHER MEMBER OF THE GROUP *(gently)*: This is a hallucination.
THERAPIST *(to Patient U)*: How do you feel about that?
PATIENT U *(smiling)*: Nice.
   *Tense silence.*
EXPERIENCED CO-THERAPIST: This is nothing unusual. This can happen. Actually, we, the therapists, represent mothers of this group. It is not surprising that you can see your mother in the therapist.

> *Another group member changes the subject and starts to talk about her job. Every afternoon after she finishes her job, she likes to go to the playground.*
> PATIENT U: My parents think that I could work harder *[he works part time at the family company].*
> *The group moves on to other issues, connected with sports, and how it is better not to do sports alone. Later on, the group discusses the negative symptoms of schizophrenia.*
>
> *Comment:* We believe that Patient U has developed a neurotic transference during his 3 years of treatment in the group (see Chapter 6). It was expressed in a psychotic way, stating that he can see his mother's head on the therapist's neck. Yet it was really an expression of protest against his being invited to the group. The invitation was perceived as aggressive, in a similar way to his mother's demands to work harder, even when psychotic. The therapists 'survived' and contained the aggressive transference and clarified (interpreted) the hallucination in a more acceptable form. Several months later, Patient U told the group that he preferred overweight girls (many girls treated for psychosis are overweight). He talked to his mother about his attraction to 'overweight' girls and she told him that he was not allowed to invite those girls home. This shows that the stigma is still present, and the mother cannot accept Patient U the way he is.
>
> The group members work through the stigma of their diagnosis and the loneliness that the illness brings to their lives. The therapists should carry a reality-based optimistic attitude towards the possibility of the patients' inclusion in interpersonal relations, in order to achieve higher levels of object relations, intersubjectivity and empathy towards others.

## Conclusion

Short- and intermediate-term groups are often designed as skill-training groups, including cognitive training, family support and other psychosocial interventions used in the treatment of early stages of psychosis. In the first phases of psychosis, patients gain better control and differentiation of their psychotic symptoms and their emotions, and improve their social functioning. Short-term groups improve adherence to treatment, reduce stigma and improve subjective quality of life.

Long-term group work has important short- and long-term effects on quality of life, attitude towards medication, social functioning and stigma reduction. Patients should be intrinsically motivated and well prepared for group work. They should be encouraged to stay in group therapy long enough to gain insight into the nature of their illness, to reduce feelings of stigma, and to become more confident and independent in social situations. The right time to leave the group should also be noted – patients should be encouraged to do so, and should be supported in the period after termination of group therapy. The termination phase is an important part of the group process in both types of groups. Further research on the specific therapeutic factors of intermediate- and long-term groups is needed.

## References

Addington J., Francey, S.M. and Morrison, A.P. (2006) *Working with People at High Risk of Developing Psychosis: A treatment handbook.* London: John Wiley & Sons.

Bernard, H., Burlingame, G.M., Flores, P., Green, L., et al. (2008) Clinical practice guidelines for group psychotherapy. *International Journal of Group Psychotherapy,* 58, 455–542.

Blinc Pesek, M., Mihoci, J., Perovšek Šolinc, N. and Avguštin, B. (2010) Long term groups for patients with psychosis in partial remission – Evaluation of ten years' work. *Psychiatria Danubina,* 22(1), 88–91.

Gabbard, G.O. (2005) *Psychodynamic Psychiatry in Clinical Practice,* 4th edition. Washington, D.C.: American Psychiatric Press.

Kanas, N. (1996) *Group Therapy for Schizophrenic Patients.* Washington, D.C.: American Psychiatric Press.

Kanas, N. (1999) 'Group therapy with schizophrenic and bipolar patients' (pp. 129–147) in V.L. Schermer and M. Pines (Eds), *Group Psychotherapy of the Psychoses.* London: Jessica Kingsley.

Lakeman, R. (2006) Adapting psychotherapy to psychosis. *Australian e-Journal for the Advancement of Mental Health (AeJAMH),* 5(1).

Martindale, B., Bateman, A., Crowe, M. and Margison, F. (2002) *Psychosis: Psychological Approaches and Their Effectiveness.* Bideford, UK: Gaskell.

Štrkalj-Ivezić, S. and Urlić, I. (2015) The capacity to use the group as a corrective symbiotic object in group analytic psychotherapy for patients with psychosis. *Group Analysis,* 48(3), 315–331.

Urlić, I. (2010) The group psychodynamic psychotherapy approach to patients with psychosis. *Psychiatria Danubina,* 22(1), 10–14.

Yalom, I. D. and Leszcz, M. (2005) *The Theory and Practice of Group Psychotherapy.* New York: Basic Books.

# Chapter 9

# Intimacy, love and sexuality in the psychodynamic group psychotherapy for patients with psychosis

*Branka Restek-Petrović, Nataša Orešković-Krezler*

## Introduction

The majority of therapists who treat psychosis through psychotherapy will agree that the issue of love and sexuality in patients with psychotic disorders has been disregarded and poorly studied (Škodlar and Žunter Nagy, 2009; Akhtar and Thomson, 1980). One of the reasons for this are the goals set in psychotherapy for patients with psychotic disorders – stabilising the disorder first and foremost, accepting the realities of mental illness and the need for long-term treatment, socialising patients and giving them the capacity for employment and a more or less independent life – and the fact that, when these goals are reached, therapy is often considered complete. The high cost of healthcare for patients with schizophrenia and other psychoses, and demands to rationalise these costs have led to a preference for quick therapeutic solutions. Patients who suffer from psychotic disorders therefore rarely have the chance to participate in long-term psychotherapy, where after attaining the basic goals of stabilising the disorder and socialisation, they would have the opportunity to develop their object relations and defence mechanisms, self-integration, the capacity for intimacy, and to establish stable, close relationships.

## Intimacy, love and sexuality in long-term psychosis groups

Psychodynamic group psychotherapy and its specificities, such as its realistic and democratic setting, presents a unique conceptual format not offered by other types of psychotherapy, and it is especially useful for the patient population with psychotic disorders (Gonzáles de Chávez, 2009). The patient has the opportunity in the here-and-now to meet and share therapeutic space with other patients, to establish communications with them under stable and nurturing conditions, and to share experiences and learn from them. By establishing a group matrix in a long-lasting group process (Foulkes, 1984), regressive object relations and primitive defense mechanisms become actualised and accessible to analysis and scrutiny, while the corrective emotional experience of good simbiosis in the group (Štrkalj Ivezić and Urlić, 2015; Restek-Petrović, 2008) opens the way to more mature and stable interpersonal relations.

In the long-term group psychotherapy process with psychotic patients, we have observed the creation of long-term friendships that overcame the time limits and boundaries of the group, as well as the creation of couples and long-term relationships – one of which ended in marriage and parenthood – which we shall describe in greater detail in this chapter, as well as their influence on the dynamics of other members and the group as a whole.

The creation of couples in psychodynamic group psychotherapy is mainly considered to be defensive and disturbing behaviour that represents an expression of subconscious regressive impulses. However, some authors (Grothjan, 1977; Nitsun, 2006) also recognise the positive aspects of this phenomenon, but only if they are contained and examined within the boundaries of a mature group.

In groups of schizophrenic patients, intimacy and love are rare occurrences, likely due to the described difficulties in the field of realising interpersonal relations. Here, we shall describe our experiences with long-term outpatient psychodynamic group psychotherapy, co-run by two group analysts in a once-weekly dynamic of one and a half hours.

## Clinical vignette 9.1

A group is composed of seven schizophrenic patients. Three female members and two male members of the group are high-functioning patients in phases of remission, with maintained social contacts, in the third decade of their lives, and all employed. All of them have several hospitalisations and years of illness behind them. The two other male members of the group are younger, included after the first episodes of their illness, one of whom is a withdrawn university student with barely any social contact and without sexual experience, and the other of whom, the youngest member, Patient S, is 20 years old and rebelling against authority through the use of drugs and promiscuous behaviour.

During the initial sessions, Patient S quickly dominates. He entertains the group with his anecdotes while 'provoking' the therapists with his frequent reports of attending parties at which he drinks alcohol and smokes marijuana, as well as with reports of skipping his medication. He is welcomed by the group, as he protects it from silence, the opening of deeper topics, and greater intimacy. A new rivalry soon begins to develop between Patient S and Patient Z, a student who often emphasises his intellectual achievements, which engenders the approval of other group members.

Patient S continues to monopolise the group even further. In an attempt to balance the 'younger' and 'older' parts of the group and prevent Patient S from dominating, the relatively inexperienced therapists introduce an additional younger female member. After a few sessions, she ceases to attend, and informs the therapists that she is leaving the group. During a group session, it is learned that she had begun a sexual relationship with Patient S, but that she was unable to admit this before the group. After a few months, the same situation repeats with another new female member. In the meantime, the remainder of the group becomes more active with support from the therapists, and begins to confront Patient S more often regarding his resistance to treatment. Patient S then leaves the group.

*Comment:* In this group, with a generational gap among the members, the youngest member fought for the exclusive attention of the therapists, entering into rivalries with the other young members, and openly in the group with Patient Z, while he 'chased' new female members out of the group by entering into sexual relations with them. After the recognition of this type of resistance in the group and after being confronted, Patient S left the group.

## Clinical vignette 9.2

A group of eight schizophrenic members is held in private practice. The members of the group, although included during the phase of the stabilisation of their illness, are regressive and withdrawn. The beginnings of the group are marked with the gradual establishment of contact, anxiousness with frequent silence, and the subjects of discussion are illness, symptoms, hospitalisation, fear of worsening illness, and the difficult experience of stigmatisation. Similarities are emphasised, which aids in developing cohesion.

With the establishment of cohesion, personal content is offered, and differences begin to be explored. An interpersonal conflict gradually develops between two members: a male patient (Patient M) with exceptionally rigid, obsessive defenses through which he has survived in stable remission and enjoyed success in his working and social life, but at the cost of his inability to create intimate emotional relationships; and a female patient with solid introspective qualities and the ability to express herself emotionally, but with weak social functionality even though she has high motivation for treatment. Despite the intervention of the therapists and group members, this dynamic dominates the group for a long time, disrupting the establishment of close relations, until one of the more regressive members of the group points out that the two are attracted to each other, which calms the constant conflict and enables the group to move on.

During the fifth year of the group, two new members arrive. Both were members of another group that ended, both are stable and in remission, and they included themselves into further psychotherapy at their own initiative. After a month, one of the new female members, Patient L, states that she and Patient T (an older member of the group) are in love and in a relationship.

*Session 178:* Patient L begins the session with the news that she and Patient T are in a relationship. She talks about how they sat in a café before the group and discussed how they would announce the news to the group, what they would say to the therapists, and how they would react. They talked about how their relationship would be accepted by their families, in the church community for Patient L, and among their friends. She cites the comments of her sister, with whom she lives, and her priest, who both asked her about Patient T, what he does and where he works, as if she were a child. Another member of the group asks how they imagined the reaction of the therapists, and Patient L says that she thought they would react like the others and think she was childish. She asks the group what they think. Two members express their surprise, but also their support for the couple. The others join in. The conversation turns to the reaction of the sister, who, as always, makes Patient L aware of the fact that she is ill and forces her own opinions on her. After this, the group then calls on Patient M and asks him what the situation is with his intimate relations. A familiar method of communication establishes itself – the whole group criticises Patient M, saying that he is too rational, too oriented towards work and money, and that he neglects his emotions, to which Patient M defends himself, saying that he currently does not need anyone, and has other preoccupations (his job, sports, renovating his flat, etc.).

*Comment:* The group reacts to the news of an emotional relationship between two group members by verbally expressing support, but instead of analysing this more deeply, the conversation turns away from intimate content by following an established pattern – urging the member of the group with the greatest problems with his emotions and intimate relations to defend his 'rigid position'. The therapists' attempt to lead the group back towards the subject of the creation of the couple, the reactions of their families, and the fear of the reaction of the therapist, are unsuccessful.

*Session 204:* A patient begins the session by expressing his feelings of sadness at the death of a close friend. Patient L remembers her mother's death from cancer when she was 13 years old and her father's death 3 years later. The third loss, being left by her boyfriend, caused the onset of her illness. Other group members also express their losses: the death of a father;

a younger sister's suicide attempt; and witnessing a serious car accident in which someone died. After a brief silence, Patient L states that Patient T has left her without explanation, over the telephone. They both decided to continue treatment in the group, as they are aware that they are ill. She feels sad, but also angry, because she thinks he should give reasons for the break-up. She points out that, before, she would have ended up in the hospital in such a situation. Another patient says that disappointment in love is a part of life, and that it must be accepted as such.

Patient L continues by saying that she only wants to know why Patient T left her. Patient T says nothing, his head bowed, and says that that is how he feels. Another member tells Patient L that, although it would be good to know the reason for the break-up, she should not insist because Patient T is obviously not ready to talk. This patient tells of his own experience from his youth when a girlfriend left him without a word, which affected him, causing him to put out cigarettes on his hand, and it crushed his self-confidence and affected his further relationships.

In a few further sessions, the group analyses this situation, and Patient L receives feedback on her demandingness and intrusiveness (asking Patient T to entrust her with everything – down to the tiniest details – making sure he takes his medication and forcing him into activities). The group also points out the similarity between this behaviour and that of her sister, which would usually bother Patient L.

As the group continues, numerous members have relationship issues: two members (one of which is Patient M) find girlfriends, another member encounters intense marital problems and faces a potential divorce, and another member experiences relationship problems with her boyfriend as he wants to get married while she is unready. Relationship problems are analysed in the group process. After 4 months, on Patient L's birthday, Patient T leaves a rose on her chair, which is an overture to their reconciliation. The entire group expresses its support.

Patient L and Patient T's relationship is now commented upon more openly in the group, and they are asked for their experiences when discussing relationship problems. One member introduces his girlfriend to the group, hoping that this will help him to understand her better. Patient L begins to share the intimate side of the relationship with the group; her fear of being touched by men, which hindered intimate relations, but which is now much improved since her relationship with Patient T. After a few of Patient L's such 'indiscretions' in the group, Patient T gets angry and states that he is leaving the group. During the following sessions, which Patient L attends alone, the sharing of intimate content, honesty, and the need for closeness as a necessary part of group work are discussed. After a month, Patient T returns on his own initiative and begins to be more open in the group.

*Comment:* The creation of a couple faces the group with problems in creating intimacy, but it also encourages the analysis of problems in close relationships. Break-ups are analysed in the group, emotions are contained, and the separation crisis in this case did not lead to a psychotic episode and hospitalisation. The group gave Patient T 'time out' and respected his inability to face his actions. The group gradually works over the reasons for his leaving Patient L, and confronts her with her intrusive and controlling behaviour, which represents a repetition of her sister's behaviour towards her. The solution of this relationship conflict and reconciliation is symbolised by a rose on Patient L's birthday, with the support of the entire group. In continued group sessions, the couple is more freely and openly communicative, and analyses intimate content. Experience with a couple in the group and the discussion of their problems influences two other male members of the group, who also form emotional relationships with girls (outside the group), while members who are married or in relationships discuss intimate problems. The group offers support, and confronts and analyses the problems of a group member threatened by divorce. The couple in the group often serves as a source of advice and experience relating to problems in emotional relationships.

## Clinical vignette 9.3

A group of young schizophrenic patients is a part of an early-intervention outpatient programme in a psychiatric hospital. The group is co-led by a group analyst and a psychiatry resident, with one one-hour session weekly. The group has nine members, all clinically stable but with difficulties in creating emotional relationships and social function. The length of participation in the group ranges from 3 to 8 years. After the planned departure of one group member, a new female member, Patient M, joins the group.

After a few months, Patient B announces that he and Patient M are in a relationship. From the very start, Patient B freely discusses his feelings, associations, and problems in his relationship with Patient M, as well as his experience of his mother's and brother's disapproval of the relationship, which often has paranoid dimensions. Patient M is well accepted in the group and begins to socialise with other female group members outside the group setting. With the approval of her parents, she invites the group to a barbecue and party in her garden, and all but the two most autistic members of the group attend.

In group discussion, Patient B frequently expresses his mother's opinion that the relationship is 'childish and stupid', and that it will quickly fail because ill people are not equipped for relationships or marriage. Patient B expresses bitterness and anger, and discusses other life experiences when he received disparagement and criticism from his mother, instead of approval. He also expresses suspicion that his older brother hates him and wants to kill him. Other group members frequently confront Patient B by telling him that this image of his mother is exaggerated, and cautiously suggesting that it is part of his illness, while they see his image of his brother as completely irrational. They support this with a specific experience that they witnessed in his company when Patient B interpreted his mother's request of him to put some chairs away as a personal attack. Patient M agrees, verbalising her opinion of Patient B's mother as a rough and emotionally distant woman, but one who wants the best for her son.

After 2 years, the couple announce that they are engaged. Patient M's parents announce that they are giving the young couple a flat, and they agree on a wedding date. The group gets involved in the excitement surrounding the wedding, helping them in their selection of a suit and wedding dress and in wedding preparations. When he attends the group without Patient M, Patient B shares his fear of being left at the altar, as well as his fears regarding how good he will be as a husband and potential father. The group provides Patient B with their significant support. Although all group members are invited to the wedding, two members attend, and at the end of the first session after the wedding, the couple treats the group and the therapists to wedding cake.

*Comment:* At a supervisory session, this situation is recounted and the couple's continued attendance of the group is considered. It is agreed that the potential transfer of one of them to another group will be discussed with them, and that the group will also be asked for their opinions. Patient M and Patient B express their desire to remain together in the group, which the group members unanimously support.

## Summary and reflection

The expression of intimate desires and sexuality is a personal issue, and it unfolds in a dyadic setting, separate from others, which requires appropriate limits. However, in this same intimate space, a great deal of anxiousness, tension, frustration, and occasionally hurt, disappointment, and abuse of power is experienced (Nitsun, 2006). In the group situation, the intimacy of the couple is presented and opened in a space shared with the other group members and the therapist(s) as witnesses, and the influence of the social setting represented by the group encompasses beyond the borders of the couple.

Sexual couples in the group, by definition, are an expression of resistance and regressive tendencies, and are interpreted as a challenge to authority that stems from an Oedipal situation. This is valid for sexual relationships that form between members outside the group, usually in secret, as a breach of the rule banning contact between group members outside the boundaries of the group. It is an expression of a group process that is insufficiently understood or managed. However, some authors also highlight the positive aspects of this phenomenon, but only if they are contained and analysed within the boundaries of a mature group.

Schizophrenic patients have great difficulties in social relations, and their relationships with others are burdened with heavy conflict and ambivalence. This type of patient suffers the greatest problems in intimate relationships, which typically demand the capacity to maintain the relationship across a longer period of time with a minimum of hostility, and hence stable and long-lasting emotional relationships are rare.

The relationships in Clinical vignette 9.1 function as resistance and are an expression of an unrecognised dynamic within the group and a lack of decisiveness in leading the group, as well as the poor selection of members. However, in Clinical vignettes 9.2 and 9.3, long-term emotional relationships appear within the group process, one of which ends in marriage. In the group in Clinical vignette 9.2, the creation of a couple enabled the group to solve long-lasting conflicts about intimacy that had hindered its progress. It also encouraged positive identification with the couple, and new emotional relationships were established (outside the group), while the empathic capacities and the capabilities for analysing intimate content of all members of the group were increased. The group in Clinical vignette 9.3 is a group of young, clinically stable but socially isolated patients, for whom the group represented nearly their sole social interaction outside of their immediate family. The creation of a couple within the group influenced broader socialisation and group outings that were analysed in the group. The group offered support to the couple, but also served the function of reality testing for distortions and projections in object relations.

In our experience, long-term group psychotherapy with psychotic patients demands that the therapist understands and adjusts the usual rules and technical procedures developed for non-psychotic patients, as well as adjusting the rules throughout the advancement of groups from autism towards richer interpersonal relationships and the capacity for psychological work. The creation of couples in the group most often presents a problem and a challenge for therapists and the entire group, but in a mature and functional group, it can be a valuable contribution to the group as a whole in its mirroring and observational function as a witness to intimate relations, thus contributing to a potentially reconstructive social process (Nitsun, 2006).

## References

Akhtar, S. and Thomson, J.A. (1980) Schizophrenia and sexuality: Review and a report of twelve unusual cases. *Journal of Clinical Psychiatry*, 41(4):134–142.
Foulkes, S.H. (1984) *Therapeutic Group Analysis*. London: Karnac Books.

Gonzáles de Chávez, M. (2009) 'Group psychotherapy and schizophrenia' in Y.O. Alanen, M. Gonzáles de Chávez, A-L.S. Silver and B. Martindale (Eds), *Psychotherapeutic Approaches to Schizophrenia Psychoses.* London: Routledge.

Grothjan, M. (1977) *Art and Technique of Analytic Group Psychotherapy.* New York: Jason Aronson.

Nitsun, M. (2006) *The Group as an Object of Desire.* London: Routledge.

Restek-Petrović, B. (2008) 'Grupna psihoterapija psihoza u ambulantnim uvjetima' ['Group psychotherapy of psychosis for outpatients'] in E. Klain (Ed), *Grupna Analiza: Analitička grupna psihoterapija [Group Analysis: Analytical group psychotherapy].* Zagreb: Medicinska naklada.

Škodlar, B. and Žunter Nagy, M. (2009) Sexuality and psychosis. *Psychiatria Danubina,* 21(1), 111–116.

Štrkalj Ivezić, S. and Urlić, I. (2015) The capacity to use the group as a corrective symbiotic object in group analytic psychotherapy for patients with psychosis. *Group Analysis,* 48, 315–331.

# Chapter 10

# The ontology and phenomenology of dreaming in psychosis

## A group-analytic approach with a neuropsychological perspective

*Anastassios Koukis*

## Introduction

This chapter[1] will continue discussion of the psychoanalytic view that patients suffering from psychosis fail to dream, and will support the idea that group analysis can help people with psychosis to reconstruct their ability to dream, thereby contributing to their therapy. It will also demonstrate that the deficit of dreaming in psychosis is on the phenomenological or manifest-content dream level, rather than on the ontological or latent-content dream level, and will briefly indicate the directions in which the psychoanalytic and group-analytic investigation of this deficit should go, with the help of neuroscientific research.

Freud (1900) believed that dreaming is a psychotic-like process in neurotic and psychotic patients alike, and that its ontology, common to both, is to depict the archaic fantasy of the primal scene. The only difference between neurotic and psychotic dreaming lies in the fact that neurotic patients are able to transform the ontological substratum of dreams, i.e., the primal scene conceived as a purely sensuous experience, into a phenomenology based on refined imagery, emotional expressiveness and rich symbolism, with mild representational distortions in a normal hallucinatory way. In contrast, patients with psychosis either lack the ability to dream altogether, like those with schizophrenia – because their unconscious is de-invested of representations of thing – or, like patients with paranoia, they produce dreams in which the phenomenological elements are highly distorted due to their deeper hallucinatory character (Freud, 1911, 1917, 1918). Leaving aside the role of the primal scene fantasy and systematic exploration of psychotic dreaming, Freud conceived neurotic dreams mainly as a phenomenological product whose sole ontological foundation was the neurotic subject's repressed Oedipal desires (Freud, 1900).

Klein (1935, 1940) restated the value of representing the fantasy of the primal scene in dreams as being initially normal in both neurotic and psychotic persons. The evolution of dreaming from representing parental intercourse in a persecuting way (paranoid–schizoid position) to representing it in a way that indicates acceptance of the parents' symbolic death (depressive position) marks the transition from psychotic dreams to dreaming proper.

For Bion (1967, 1992), dreams are the inner projections of visual images of a good enough mother (Freud's 'thing') and of the fantasy of the primal scene as it evolved from a sensory/ontological experience into an 'ideogram' of the parental union (phenomenological level), and marks the transition from the oral–sadistic stage to the paranoid–schizoid position and the depressive position as a mature Oedipal situation (Bion, 1992, pp. 52, 64). He sees dreaming as the ability to digest mentally the need for the breast as real day and night and consists of resuckling at the breast on a symbolic level by projecting visual images on the dream screen or as suckling by recounting dreams in a psychoanalytic session. Patients with psychosis fail to dream because they depict the primal scene solely as a sensual and fragmentary experience. This is a result of the hallucinated suckling they received from a mother conceived as a 'dead' object inside them, as a result of which they continuously desire (and retain a strong memory of) the breast as real thing. This is why they can only visualise the mother in the form of fragmented images that persecute them during the paranoid–schizoid position on which they are fixated. People with psychosis fragment the images in their dreams (this is a way of avoiding entrance to the depressive position by splitting it), through excessive projective identifications against themselves and the object inside them (Bion, 1992). Psychotic dreams are only 'invisible–visual hallucinations' (Bion, 1967, p. 96) or projective identifications turned against the therapist or the group through their recounting. Bion (1967, 1992) does not rule out the possibility that psychotic patients in psychoanalysis could dream to some extent, by depicting the primal scene in a somewhat articulated phenomenology.

Foulkes (1964) argues that dreams constitute narcissistic encapsulations and are therefore by nature psychotic processes in either their neurotic or psychotic form. Dreaming by patients suffering from neurosis or psychosis can become a healthy activity only on condition that it is produced in the form of group dreams in a group-analytic group by expressing the quality of the dynamics in its matrix based on a number of group phenomena and factors, such as communication, condenser phenomena, mirror reactions, transposition, etc. The phenomenology of this group communication, as expressed on the intermediate-level/phase of the group's bodily and mental images (Freud's anal–sadistic stage or Klein's paranoid–schizoid position) and principally on the third current level/phase (Freud's phallic stage or Klein's depressive position) constitutes – unlike the ontology of the group as manifested on its first archaic/primordial (oral–sadistic) level/phase – a dreaming process that the members' dreams depict as group dreams. Foulkes totally neglects the idea that the dreams of patients with neurosis or psychosis could, through group dreams, express the ontology of group process as an evolved fantasy of the primal scene represented by the union of therapist and group.

## Dreaming as the evolution of the fantasy of the primal scene in the group

According to the views of Klein and Bion, archaic fantasies like that of the primal scene, together with certain primordial defence mechanisms such as projection, splitting or projective identification, could be considered as constituting the primal nucleus of human sociality, of which dreaming is a basic manifestation. In this study, the role of the group in the production of dreams will be reconsidered as a representation of the fantasy of the primal scene, which helps patients with psychosis in group analysis to reconstitute some degree of their ability to dream.

### Introductory remarks

The quality of dreaming by patients with psychosis or neurosis is successively articulated in the form of group dreams (Foulkes, 1964), and is correlated with the progressive evolution of the group from representing the imaginary union of therapist and group as a fantasy of the primal scene to representing the union of the conductor and the group as a highly symbolic idea of the parental couple. This evolution follows, continuously and in a spiral form, that of the group from its oral–sadistic stage to the paranoid–schizoid position and the depressive position, and of the therapist from a directive archaic father figure (leader) to a symbolic father figure (conductor), trust in whom reveals the group's pre-eminent maturity as described by Foulkes (1964). Mirror phenomena and especially matrix have also given the group a 'capacity for reverie' style that characterises the good enough mother in particular, and is lacking in the psychotic patient (Bion, 1992, p. 53), while also helping the therapist, who needs to avoid any related interpretations.

Here, briefly, is the way in which two patients with psychosis, Patient S and Patient G,[2] were able to dream properly by depicting in their dreams the fantasy of the primal scene and its evolution towards the idea of combined parents. This process was assisted significantly by other (mainly neurotic or borderline) patients who recounted their dreams within a dreaming matrix. The patients were members of a heterogeneous once-a-week group-analytic group. They entered the group after about 3 and 4 years respectively of once-a-week individual psychotherapy. Patient S is a social worker, 26 years old, who lives alone. Her symptoms included schizophrenic pathology, such as hearing voices and believing that people kept talking about her on television. She entered the group as a new member and left it after about 6 years of therapy, when her symptoms receded considerably and her ability to dream had been significantly reconstituted. Patient G, also 26 years old, a mathematician, who also lives alone, was a founding member of the group. He suffered from acute paranoid psychosis. He usually imagined that he was God and was hospitalised twice. Through his individual and group therapy and medication, the symptoms progressively receded. There were no further hospitalisations, the ability to dream was sufficiently reconstructed and Patient G was able to bid a successful farewell to the group after about 8 years of therapy.

## First stage

During the first stage, which lasted from 6 months to about 1 year, the patients' initial recounted (mainly individual) dreams indicated that the fantasy of the primal scene, and of the group conceived as such, was either hidden in dreams that had all the features of delirium (Patient G's dream), or was depicted in the form of another primary fantasy such as that of the mother with the penis (Patient S's dream). Both dreams were somewhat similar to many dreams recounted by other members. In these dreams, the primal scene was presented as totally split, in the sense that the maternal body was depicted as a total of paternal penises (usually symbolised by snake images) and infants (symbolised by babies) which are 'dead' (Patient J's dream). All dreams reveal that the primal scene cannot be represented because the patients' mirroring in the maternal object/group is absent in this phase due to their fixation in the oral–sadistic stage/primordial level of the group.

This is illustrated by one of the first group dreams of a borderline patient, Patient C, in which women and men, including the group therapist, are depicted without eyes. The recounting of dreams of this kind constitutes projective identifications that aim to stir up the corresponding primeval/psychotic experience which, at least in its initial phase, the group inevitably encompasses.

PATIENT G: I dreamed I was God.
PATIENT J: A snake was threatening me, and lots of babies and dead people.
PATIENT S: My mother was naked with a penis in front.
PATIENT C: I saw men and women who have no eyes and that our therapist had no eyes.

## Second stage

During the second stage, which lasted from 1 to 2 years, the dreams of the patients suffering from psychosis recounted in the group, as either individual productions or more often as group dreams, evidently emerged from a first mirroring of the dreaming person with the group conceived as a good enough dreaming process. The dreams mainly express paranoid anxiety (paranoid–schizoid position), but the projective identification with the group is now much milder. It can then be contained by the group and in turn supports the function of the group as container (Friedman, 2000).

The fantasy of the primal scene has begun to be represented specifically in a persecutory way, either in the form of the father's or mother's penis (symbolised by a knife) that tries to penetrate the patient from behind (Patient S's first dream), or as the fantasy of the mother with the penis in a milder, more effeminate form (Patient S's second dream). It can also take the form of the union of the conductor conceived as Christ and the group as Church within a state that continues to express delirium and in which the patient is still God (Patient G's dream).

These dreams do not differ in content from the dreams reported by other patients during the same period. A dream reported by Patient M, a neurotic patient suffering from panic attacks, expressed the paranoid–schizoid position depicted as an attack against the patient by dogs (representing the conductor), in which the primal scene is imperceptibly represented by the union of the conductor/dogs and the patient. The dreams of non-psychotic patients, however, differ from psychotic dreams in terms of the higher level of their representational quality and emotional tone, the finer selection of dream symbols, and the sophisticated use of language either in the process of dreaming itself or in its narration.

PATIENT S: I was sleeping on my stomach; a knife comes from above and pierces me.

PATIENT G: I enter a church. Suddenly Christ appears. 'I am God too,' I say to him.

PATIENT S: It was in a place sort of like where the group meets. Suddenly a naked woman appeared; she had a plastic vulva and inside this plastic thing was a penis, also plastic.

PATIENT M: A pack of dogs was coming toward me.

### Third stage

During the third stage, in which the depressive position continues to develop uninterruptedly in the group in negotiation with the paranoid–schizoid position, the dreams reported by the patients suffering from psychosis seem to possess a number of neurotic features, thus indicating the patients' first sufficient, although unstable, entrance into the depressive position. Dreams are of a finer group character and are narrated through projective identification in the sense of a good enough communication. The patient is now better mirrored in the group and is mirrored by it more effectively. The fantasy of the mother with the penis seems to be sufficiently repressed, and this is helped by dreaming itself, by the mother allowing her penis to fall off (Patient S's first dream). The primal scene, although it is still homosexual in nature as a union of two men – the father and the phallic mother – indicates the patient's first attempt to achieve the parents' symbolic death by using the depressive position, although in a wild archaic way (Patient S's second dream). In other cases, the primal scene is symbolised in dreams as the marriage of the person's parents (or the 'marriage' of the conductor and the group), even though the couple either cannot be clearly discerned (Patient G's first dream) or it is the friend's father, not the patient's father, who marries the patient's mother (Patient G's second dream) or later as a marriage of his parents (or group and conductor) within the group, as symbolised by a carriage in a way that indicates to some extent the parents' symbolic death (Patient G's third dream).

Again, these dreams lack the emotional quality and the symbolic and imaginative plasticity that characterises the dreams of neurotic patients, indicating the latter's more stable entrance into the depressive position. For example, in Patient M's dreams, the primal scene is symbolised by her own wedding linked with her mourning for the symbolic death of her parents (or group and conductor); in psychotic dreams any indication of mourning is totally absent.

PATIENT S: I saw a naked woman; in place of her pudenda, was a penis that fell off.

PATIENT G: I'd gone to a wedding, but couldn't figure out who the newlyweds were.

PATIENT G: I dreamt that the father of my friend married my mother.

PATIENT G: I saw a dead man, maybe my father. But then everything was like a wedding. It was inside a carriage and many of you were there.

PATIENT S: I was in an ancient theatre. It was dark and on the stage there were two posts on which were the heads of two men; the heads were alive. Then the heads died.

PATIENT M: My parents have died. I'm preparing for the funeral and crying but suddenly I am to be married and getting ready to go and see about a wedding dress.

## Conclusions and remarks about future neuroscience research

Dreaming in psychosis can evolve into dreaming with neurotic features in a heterogeneous group-analytic group, thereby making a decisive contribution to the patient's therapy. This is because, like dreaming in neurosis, psychotic dreaming follows and expresses the group's evolution (conceived as the union of therapist and group) from the pre-Oedipal primordial/ontological level (oral–sadistic stage and paranoid–schizoid position), on which it represents the primal scene as a sensual experience, to the final current phenomenological Oedipal level (depressive position) representing the primal scene as depicting an ideal parental couple according to the views of Klein (1935, 1940) and Bion (1967, 1992). This group approach and its impact on dreaming were totally ignored by Foulkes (1964).

These conclusions, however, should be accepted with some reservations. In fact, patients with psychosis do not dream in a regular/neurotic way (Freud, 1911, 1917, 1918; Bion, 1967, 1992), and we are still a long way from being able to help them to dream in the way of patients with neurosis. Although the latter's dreams also express the primal scene on the ontological level, the phenomenology of neurotic patients' dreams is much more sophisticated in the use of emotion, language, imagery and symbolism than that of dreams by patients with psychosis.

What, then, is the factor missing in the process of transforming the ontology of psychotic dreaming into the phenomenology of a good enough neurotic content? The answer to this question should not rely solely on psychoanalytic investigation. Neuroscientific research has verified Freud's (1900) views of a core common to dreaming and psychosis (Gottesmann, 2006; Scarone, et al., 2008). Further extension of this research would be of great help in elucidating the above question.

To what extent, for example, is the lack of any phenomenological articulation of psychotic dreaming related to an enduring memory of and desire for a real breast (Bion, 1992), and in what respects are psychotic memory and desire the result of the defective inhibition of dream memory (Kelly, 1998)? Do they represent a failure of the superior temporal and inferior parietal deactivation (Fletcher, et al., 1998)? Or, should we elaborate on the hypothesis that, in the case of psychotic patients, some potential memories have not been eliminated before being stored in the long-term memory, thus resulting in inefficient memory processing linked with reduced cerebral metabolism in frontal areas due to the reductions of synaptic density caused by excessive axonal pruning (Hoffman and Dobscha, 1989; Feinberg, 1982–1983)? Or should we link the lack of imagery in psychotic dreaming to the fact that people with psychosis develop hallucinatory activity during waking hours – which is also a dreamlike activity (Bion, 1992) – instead of during rapid eye movement (REM) sleep, owing to serotonin depletion (Zarcone, et al., 1975; Dement, et al., 1969)? In addition, could any phenomenological deficiency in psychotic dreaming be interpreted as a deficiency in the mirror-neuron system (Rizzolatti and Craighero, 2004)? Could the mirror-neuron system explain the fundamental role played by the fantasy of the primal scene – as based primarily on the mirroring between parents and child or between the group members/children and the group/mother and/or the conductor/father– in the formation of dreams in psychotic and neurotic patients alike?

These are some of the basic questions that future psychoanalytic and group-analytic research should investigate through neuroscience, to ascertain whether or not the findings reported here can be further validated and thereby opening new perspectives in understanding psychosis and in approaching it more effectively through psychotherapy.

## Notes

1   This chapter is modified from a version already published in the journal *Psychology Research* (David Publishing Company), and in the book *On Group Analysis and Beyond* (Karnac Books).
2   Although all group members in this chapter are not given their names, the clinical material related to them is real. I would like to thank them all for giving me permission to publish their stories.

## References

Bion, W.R. (1967) *Second Thoughts*. London: Heinemann.
Bion, W.R. (1992) *Cogitations*. London: Karnac.
Dement, W., Zarcone, V.P. Jr, Ferguson, J., Cohen, H., et al. (1969) 'Some parallel findings in schizophrenic patients and serotonin depleted cats' (pp. 775–811) in S. Sankar (Ed), *Schizophrenia: Current concepts and research*. Hicksville: PJD Publications.
Feinberg, I. (1982–1983) Schizophrenia: Caused by a fault in programmed synaptic elimination during adolescence? *Journal of Psychiatric Research*, 17(4), 319–334.

Fletcher, P.C., McKenna, P.J., Frith, C.D., Grasby, P.M., et al. (1998) Brain activations in schizophrenia during a graded memory task studied with functional neuroimaging. *Archives of General Psychiatry*, 55, 1001–1008.

Foulkes, S.H. (1964) *Therapeutic Group Analysis*. London: Allen & Unwin.

Freud, S. (1900) *The Interpretation of Dreams. S.E., IV-V*. London: Hogarth.

Freud, S. (1911) *Psycho-Analytic Notes on an Autobiographical Account of a Case of Paranoia (dementia paranoides). S.E., XII*. London: Hogarth.

Freud, S. (1917). *A Metapsychological Supplement to the Theory of Dreams. S.E., XIV.* London: Hogarth.

Freud, S. (1918). *From the History of an Infantile Neurosis. S.E., XVII*. London: Hogarth.

Friedman, R. (2000) The interpersonal containment of dreams in group psychotherapy: A contribution to the work with dreams in a group. *Group Analysis*, 33(2), 221–233.

Gottesmann, C. (2006) The dreaming sleep stage: A new neurobiological model of schizophrenia? *Neuroscience*, 140(4), 1105–1115.

Hoffman, R.E. and Dobscha, S.K. (1989) Critical pruning and the development of schizophrenia: A computer model. *Schizophrenia Bulletin*, 15(3), 477–490.

Kelly, P.H. (1998) Defective inhibition of dream event memory formation: A hypothesized mechanism in the onset and progression of symptoms of schizophrenia. *Brain Research Bulletin*, 46(3), 189–197.

Klein, M. (1935/1998) 'A contribution to the psychogenesis of manic-depressive states' (pp. 262–289) in M. Klein (Ed), *Love, Guilt and Reparation and other Works: 1921–1945,* 2nd edition. London: Vintage.

Klein, M. (1940/1998). 'Mourning and its relation to manic-depressive states' (pp. 344–369) in M. Klein (Ed), *Love, Guilt and Reparation and other Works: 1921–1945,* 2nd edition. London: Vintage.

Rizzolatti, G. and Craighero, L. (2004) The mirror-neuron system. *Annual Review of Neuroscience*, 27, 169–192.

Scarone, S., Manzone, M.L., Gambini, O., Kantzas, I., et al. (2008) The dream as a model for psychosis: An experimental approach using bizarreness as a cognitive marker. *Schizophrenia Bulletin*, 34(3), 515–522.

Zarcone, V.P. Jr, Azumi, K., Dement, W., Gulevitc, G., et al. (1975) REM phase deprivation and schizophrenia II. *Archives of General Psychiatry*, 32, 1431–1436.

# Chapter 11

# Psychoeducation as a specific group psychotherapy intervention for patients with schizophrenia

*Slađana Štrkalj Ivezić*

## Introduction

Psychoeducation is a systemic, didactic–psychotherapeutic intervention, aimed to facilitate both an understanding and a personally responsible handling of illness, and a support for those affected by the disorder (Bäuml, et al., 2006). Most patients with schizophrenia do not accept the biological concept of the disease, and this may result in abandoning treatment. Therefore, psychobiosocial concepts of illness, based on stress vulnerability theory and information shared in a therapeutic culture of recovery and empowerment, should be accepted as a basic principle in any kind of information about the illness, for patients as well as for their families.

Meta-analysis (Xia, Merinder and Belgamwar, 2011) has confirmed the efficacy of psychoeducation in decreasing relapse rates and frequency of hospitalisation, and in increasing medication adherence, but, paradoxically, it does not increase insight into illness. Studies offer contradictory findings concerning the influence of insight into illness on treatment outcomes. On the one hand, higher insight is related to good outcome (Lysaker, Roe and Yano, 2007); but on the other hand, a higher level of insight is associated with a number of negative outcomes, such as: low self-esteem (Corrigan, et al., 2010), higher probability of developing depressive mood (Drake, et al., 2004), feelings of hopelessness (Yanos, et al., 2008; Corrigan, et al., 2010), and lower quality of life (Staring, et al., 2009). The paradoxical results can be explained by the meaning that a person attributes to the diagnosis (Lysaker, Roe and Yano, 2007). Many patients feel that a diagnosis of schizophrenia inevitably implies a poor prognosis and poor outcome. They therefore believe that there is no hope for them to recover or to lead a satisfying life (Deegan, 1988).

Studies have confirmed that associations of insight with depression, low quality of life, and negative self-esteem are moderated by stigma (Staring, et al., 2009). Hence, patients with insight who do not perceive much stigmatisation seem to perform better across various outcome parameters. About half of patients treated for schizophrenia suffer internalised stigma (Brohan, et al., 2010), with its numerous negative consequences such as: low self-esteem, helplessness, loss of hope, low quality of life, increased risk of depression, higher level of psychopathology (Mak and Wu, 2006; Lysaker, Roe and Yano, 2007), loss of self-respect, problems with dignity, fear, shame and guilt (Corrigan, 1998; Van Brakel, 2006), and identity change (Yanos, et al., 2008). Studies have shown that the impact of insight into illness in schizophrenia on self-confidence, hope and functioning depends on the degree to which a person internalises stigmatising attitudes about the disease (Lysaker, Roe and Yano, 2007).

Up-to-date knowledge concerning the association of insight and self-stigma, and its connection with the process of transformation of identity in which a person loses his/her existing or desired identity and adopts a stigmatising view of him/herself, implies the need to find effective methods, such as psychoeducation, in order to improve insight into illness. In order to prevent internalised stigma causing a negative transformation of the self, psychoeducation should integrate educational, psychotherapeutic and sociotherapeutic elements. Educational goals include increasing knowledge about the disease and its treatment and recovery, and acquiring basic competency for well-informed and self-competent decisions about treatment options. Patients are taught about medication, recognising symptoms of illness including the early signs of deterioration, building supportive networks, improving family communication, developing the skills needed for everyday life, coping with stress, anxiety and stigma, and preventing self-stigmatisation – all of which are important for recovery. An indispensable part of information about the disease should be the key message that recovery is possible.

Psychotherapeutic goals include: working through the psychological reactions to the diagnosis of mental illness and the stigma of mental illness; assigning individual meanings to symptoms; understanding the illness in the context of personal experience; avoiding negative self-concept change; transforming identity as patient toward identity as person; rejecting stereotypes of mental illness as personally relevant; and building effective coping skills for stigma and discrimination. The psychological aspects of psychoeducation include: emotions related to the diagnosis, stigma and discrimination; anticipation of rejection; isolation from people; depression and suicidal tendencies; identity change; and the experience of loss. Work with self-esteem and self-respect refers to working through emotions of shame, guilt, helplessness, hopelessness, anxiety, depression and anger. Sociotherapy goals include: working with attitudes about the illness and treatment, including medication and psychosocial treatment; improving skills needed for efficient coping with stigma and discrimination; and interpersonal functioning. Expectations from effective psychoeducation include: overcoming the idea of illness as catastrophic event; insight into the disease associated with empowerment and prevention of self-stigma; acceptance of a person's identity as opposed to the identity of patient; and prevention of relapse, including a reduced need for hospitalisation and increased adherence to treatment.

Information about the disease has limited impact on attitudes towards the disease (Corrigan, et al., 2001). Therefore, education about the disease within the psychotherapeutical framework should provide dialogue about the personal meaning of diagnosis and symptoms, as well as help in rejecting the stereotypes and stigma that are associated with mental illness (Štrkalj-Ivezić, 2013). The patient in this integrated model of psychoeducation has a chance to understand the symptoms of illness on a personal level in the context of his/her life, to understand the meanings of symptoms on a psychological level, and to acquire an empowering experience that makes it possible to affect the outcome of the illness and to change the negative image of the self, as caused by transformation of the self after the diagnosis of mental illness (Štrkalj Ivezić, 2013). If implemented correctly, psychoeducation provides a powerful tool, with the potential to redirect the course of the illness toward the path of recovery.

## Psychoeducation in the framework of group psychotherapy

The group represents a micro-social system, encouraging the process of redefinition of the self, and is therefore particularly suitable for working through topics related to attitudes toward the disease, stigma and identity, as well as working through emotions. Kanas (1986, 1991, 1993, 1996, 1999) has proven the effectiveness of group psychotherapy, where goals included patient education about the disease, improvement in coping with the symptoms of the disease, testing of reality, and interpersonal communication. A number of qualitative studies have identified the importance of acceptance, hope, redefinition of self, empowerment, social support, and establishment of meaning and purpose in life, for recovery from mental illness (Smith, et al., 2000; Andresen, Caputi and Oades, 2006). In this sense, group psychotherapy, with its therapeutical factors such as universality, acceptance, cohesion, hope and altruism (Yalom and Leszcz, 2005; González de Chávez, 2009) facilitates the recovery process. Furthermore, our clinical experience with the model of psychoeducation presented here confirms its effectiveness in reduction of self-stigma (Štrkalj-Ivezić, Sesar and Mužinić, 2017). This model considers psychoeducation as a group psychotherapy that combines educational, psychosocial and psychotherapeutic goals that are mutually intertwined in the majority of group sessions.

Psychoeducation as a group psychotherapy should be recommended to all patients with a diagnosis of schizophrenia, especially those who have difficulty accepting the diagnosis, do not adhere to treatment, and are at risk of self-stigmatisation. Psychoeducation is best begun immediately after the establishment of diagnosis, during hospital treatment or shortly after discharge. However, education can begin at any time, even after many years of illness and/or during each recurrence of symptoms. Psychoeducation is best provided in the stabilisation phase of the disease.

It is recommended that psychoeducation in group psychotherapy be carried out with a minimum of 12 sessions, but for some patients, longer durations may be required. If the goals are dedicated exclusively to information about the disease and treatment in order to help patients make decisions about their treatment, the duration may be less than 12 sessions. However, when the goals are more psycho-therapeutical, such as the emotional aspects of diagnosis, stigma and attitudes toward the disease, as well as the psychological meaning of symptoms, and insight, longer durations are needed. The participation of persons having recovered from schizophrenia in one of the sessions has proved useful, especially for the restoration of hope, the facilitation of recovery, and the fight against self-stigmatisation.

All meetings should have a similar structure. Before joining the group, all patients are informed that education about the disease helps them to learn to use the information obtained in the group to maintain their health and to prevent repeat episodes of illness. Members are advised of the list of topics that will be covered during a minimum of 12 meetings of the group. Members are also told that regular visits to meetings are expected, and that each meeting lasts 60 to 90 minutes, and combines didactic–educational elements such as a short presentation of inform-ation about the illness, with interactive discussion. Information about the disease is presented in a way that opens up possibilities of recovery, as opposed to the perspective of chronicity. Particular attention is paid to the discussion of myths about mental illness. After a short informal introduction, which is used to create a good atmosphere, the group begins by summarising the key messages from the previous meeting, with the possibility of further questions, comments and provi-sion of additional clarification of content from the previous group. Educational topics to be treated at the meeting are normally agreed upon in the previous group session. Prior to the presentation by the therapist of up-to-date information on the topic selected for discussion, personal knowledge, attitudes and emotional reactions to the topic are stimulated and discussed. The goals are to uncover the attitudes, emotions and transformation of identity connected with the illness.

In the next step, the therapist provides professional and scientific information on the educational topic, discusses misconceptions and stigmatised attitudes, and facilitates working through attitudes and emotions with the group. The therapist stimulates open discussion and interaction between members, and before the end of the session summarises the information discussed in the group in terms of knowledge, attitudes and emotional reactions. Information about the disease given by the therapist is based on information in accordance with up-to-date knowledge about the disease, its symptoms, treatment and outcome. The psychobiosocial model of disease, free of stigmatised attitude, is a basic requirement for providing education about the illness. Recovery and empowerment principles are built mainly on the presented information. For educational purposes, in the explanation of each topic, the therapist may use data obtained from a group member, examples from clinical practice, or from the literature. In the further course of the group process, the therapist stimulates discussion about the connection between given information on the disease and its treatment to group members' personal experiences, and thus stimulates additional questions and gives further clarification if required.

The personal experiences of group members with symptoms of illness, including emotional reactions and attitudes, are especially important, because this is the way in which patients connect information with their experience, helping them to test reality, achieve insight into the illness, recognise early symptoms of disease, reduce pathological behaviour stemming from symptoms, and to change their attitudes toward the disease (rejecting cultural stereotypes about mental illness as relevant to them). Educational content is presented in a manner that encourages and facilitates open dialogue. A clear message is transmitted to all members of the group that they are experts on the basis of their experience, and that their contributions to the group discussion, related to sharing knowledge, attitudes, and emotional experience, is extremely valuable and beneficial to all members of the group, including the therapist.

Based on the presented information and discussion during the group session, at the end of the session concluding remarks are proposed by the group members and/or by the therapist. If recommendations are proposed by the therapist, he/she will seek acceptance from group members. Patients are motivated to return to the next meeting if they keep some questions until then. Conclusions always favour empowerment, recovery and nonstigmatised attitudes, and they encourage the use of the knowledge, attitudes and experiences gained in the group in real-life situations.

For less skilled therapists who are not group psychotherapists, a more structured group discussion that focuses primarily on educational objectives related to information about the illness and attitudes is recommended. In such a group, emotional experience is generally not worked through.

## The therapist as conductor of the psychoeducational group

For the therapist in psychoeducation group psychotherapy, it is essential that he/she has accepted the psychobiosocial model of illness and the principles of recovery as treatment goals, has knowledge of psychological theories related to the understanding of psychosis, and is able to reject stereotypes of mental illness. It is desirable that the therapist has experience in their own work of patients recovering, even when their mental state is declared chronic. Authentic belief that the patient can become more competent and have hope for the future is a basic requirement for work with a group of such patients.

All interventions in the group are carried out in an atmosphere of clear care and interest for patients' difficulties. The therapist nurtures an atmosphere of trust, acceptance, respect and optimism, taking care that anxiety levels are tolerable for group members. Special care is devoted to avoiding high emotional arousal, because it is associated with a high risk of psychotic symptoms. The therapist must take into account the capabilities of group members for tolerance of anxiety and, in accordance with the situation in a group, must reduce anxiety and close every group session in a calming atmosphere. Flexibility is required of the therapist due to the tendency of the group to oscillate from one topic to another, which may not be related to the selected educational theme. The therapist should encourage discussion about the topic in a way that allows for free exchange of thoughts and emotions. Depending on the skills of the therapist, group work may fluctuate more towards educational (information sharing), or psychotherapeutical (related to personal emotional experiences with the disease and the discovery of the psychological meaning of symptoms).

In groups with psychotherapeutic goals, patients should be given the opportunity to work through emotions related to diagnosis and stigma of mental illness. The therapist must be prepared for the occurrence of depression after the insight into illness in some of the patients. He/she must understand the reasons for this depression and help the patient to overcome the depression, as well as using members of the group to help the patient. The most common interventions in the group include education and counselling, confrontation with reality, and clarification by linking symptoms with personal experience (for example, the idea of persecution can be connected to trust difficulties). The therapist should pay special attention to stigma and self-stigma. Viewing patients positively, through the perspective of recovery rather than through cultural stereotypes, can help to combat the negative consequences of stigma (Štrkalj-Ivezić, 2013). The following topics may be worked through in psychotherapeutic groups:

- individual and personal symptoms of members' psychotic disorders;
- member's views on the possible causes of psychosis;
- recovery and individual goals of treatment;
- stress and anxiety;
- comprehensive treatment of schizophrenia/psychosis;
- self-esteem and identity;
- stigma and self-stigma.

## Conclusion

For psychoeducation as a psychotherapeutic intervention, it is important to obtain informed consent for treatment and to establish a treatment alliance, which is standard procedure for each patient. Psychoeducation as described here is a form of supportive group psychotherapy combining educational elements (information about the illness, its treatment, and stigma), psychotherapy (working through emotional response to the disease/diagnosis and stigma, and understanding the psychological meaning of symptoms of the disease as a part of personal experience), and working with attitudes toward illness (stigma and self-stigma), as well as sociotherapeutic approaches such as promoting skills building and successfully coping with stress. The principles of empowerment and recovery are part of this method, with respect to all the previously mentioned aspects.

Educational, psychotherapeutic and sociotherapeutic elements including work on stigma and self-stigma are intertwined in every group session and are processed within the therapist and group members' interactions. The basic principles of psychoeducation include the psychobiosocial model of illness, empowerment and recovery goals, and fighting against the stigma and discrimination associated with mental illness. Special attention is paid to work on the rejection of stereotypes of mental illness, and the generation of insight into illness, which is connected with good outcomes.

Psychoeducation is not a series of lectures about the symptoms of mental illness and its treatments.

Rather, it is a psychotherapeutic process that includes open discussion about the symptoms of the disease, the psychological and social consequences of the disease, and understanding the disease in the context of personal life. Psychoeducation also affects the decision-making process in choosing beneficial treatment. It helps to restore patients' confidence in their own capacity to lead life in a productive and satisfactory manner. To create a successful programme, one needs to integrate knowledge of psychodynamic psychotherapy, group psychotherapy, public and internalised stigma, rehabilitation based on principles of recovery, and long-term experience of working with patients with a diagnosis of psychosis treated in rehabilitation programmes and psychotherapy. Up-to-date knowledge regarding the connection between insight and self-stigma and the process of transformation of identity, implies the need to find effective methods, such as the psychoeducation model presented here, in order to achieve insight into illness connected with a low level of internalised stigma and therefore to prevent any negative transformation of the self.

## References

Andresen, R., Caputi, P. and Oades, L. (2006) The stages of recovery instrument: Development of a measure of recovery from serious mental illness. *Australian and New Zealand Journal of Psychiatry*, 40, 972–980.

Bäuml, J., Fröböse, T., Kraemer, S., Rentrop, M., et al. (2006) Psychoeducation: A basic psychotherapeutic intervention for patients with schizophrenia and their families. *Schizophrenia Bulletin*, 1, S1–S9.

Brohan, E., Elgie, R., Sartorius, N. and Thornicroft, G. (2010) GAMIAN-Europe study group: Self-stigma, empowerment and perceived discrimination among people with schizophrenia in 14 European countries: the GAMIAN-Europe study. *Schizophrenia Research*, 122, 232–238.

Corrigan, P.W. (1998) The impact of stigma on severe mental illness. *Cognitive and Behavioral Practice*, 5, 201–222.

Corrigan, P.W., Morris, S., Larson, J., Rafacz, J., et al. (2010) Self-stigma and coming out about one's mental illness. *American Journal of Community Psychology*, 38, 259–275.

Corrigan, P.W., River L.P., Lundin R.K., Penn, D.L., et al. (2001) Three strategies for changing attributions about severe mental illness. *Schizophrenia Bulletin*, 27(2), 187–195.

Deegan, P.E. (1988) Recovery: The lived experience of rehabilitation. *Psychosocial Rehabilitation Journal*, 11, 11–19.

Drake, R.J., Pickles, A., Bentall, R.P., Kinderman, P., et al. (2004) The evolution of insight, paranoia and depression during early schizophrenia. *Psychological Medicine*, 34(2), 285–292.

González de Chávez, M. (2009) 'Group psychotherapy and schizophrenia' (pp. 251–266) in Y.O. Alanen, M. González de Chávez, A-L.S. Silver, B. Martindale (Eds), *Psychotherapeutic Approaches to Schizophrenic Psychoses: Past, present and future.* New York: Routledge.

Kanas, N. (1986) Group therapy with schizophrenics: A review of controlled studies. *International Journal of Group Psychotherapy,* 36, 339–351.

Kanas, N. (1991) Group therapy with schizophrenic patients: A short-term, homogeneous approach. *International Journal of Group Psychotherapy,* 41, 33–48.

Kanas, N. (1993) Group psychotherapy with bipolar patients: A review and synthesis. *International Journal of Group Psychotherapy,* 43(3), 321–33.

Kanas, N. (1996) *Group Therapy with Schizophrenic Patients.* Washington, D.C.: American Psychiatric Press.

Kanas, N. (1999) 'Group therapy with schizophrenic and bipolar patients: Integrative approaches' in V.L. Schermer and M. Pines (Eds), *Group Psychotherapy of the Psychoses.* London: Jessica Kingsley.

Lysaker, P.H., Roe, D. and Yano, P.T. (2007) Toward understanding the insight paradox: Internalized stigma moderates the association between insight and social functioning, hope, and self-esteem among people with schizophrenia spectrum disorders. *Schizophrenia Bulletin,* 33, 192–199.

Mak, W.W.S. and Wu, C.F.M. (2006) Cognitive insight and causal attribution in the development of self-stigma among individuals with schizophrenia. *Psychiatric Services,* 57(12), 1800–1802.

Smith, T.E., Hull, J.W., Israel, L.M. and Willson, D.F. (2000) Insight, symptoms, and neurocognition in schizophrenia and schizoaffective disorder. *Schizophrenia Bulletin,* 26, 193–200.

Staring, A.B.P., Van der Gaag, M., Van den Berge, M., Duivenvoorden, H.J., et al. (2009) Stigma moderates the associations of insight with depressed mood, low self-esteem, and low quality of life in patients with schizophrenia spectrum disorders. *Schizophrenia Research,* 115, 363–369.

Štrkalj-Ivezić, S. (2013) Stigma in clinical practice. *Psychiatria Danubina,* 25(2), S200–202.

Štrkalj-Ivezić, S., Sesar, M.A. and Mužinić, L. (2017) Effects of a group psychoeducation program on self-stigma, empowerment, and perceived discrimination of persons with schizophrenia. *Psychiatria Danubina,* 29(1), 66–73.

Van Brakel, V.H. (2006) Measuring health-related stigma – A literature review. *Psychology, Health and Medicine,* 11, 307–334.

Xia, J., Merinder, L.B. and Belgamwar, M.R. (2011) Psychoeducation for schizophrenia. *Schizophrenia Bulletin,* 37, 21–22.

Yalom, I. and Leszcz, M. (2005) *The Theory and Practice of Group Psychotherapy,* 5th edition. New York: Basic Books.

Yanos, P.T., Roe, D., Markus, K. and Lysaker, P.H. (2008) Pathways between internalized stigma and outcomes related to recovery in schizophrenia-spectrum disorders. *Psychiatric Services,* 59, 1437–1442.

# Chapter 12

# Groups in therapeutic communities for people suffering from psychosis

*David Kennard*

## Introduction

Groups of various types form a central part of therapeutic community theory and practice. In this chapter I will begin by briefly outlining the history of therapeutic communities, with particular reference to the care and treatment of people suffering from psychosis. The chapter will distinguish between three types of therapeutic community: psychiatric admission wards using a therapeutic community approach; settings providing 'alternative' asylum, including the Soteria model, to support people in an acute psychotic phase; and therapeutic communities supporting the rehabilitation/recovery for people with long-term psychosis. I will describe the different types and uses of groups with some clinical illustrations. Uses of groups include:

- community meetings;
- small-group therapy;
- action-based groups (e.g., art, psychodrama);
- task groups (e.g., cleaning, gardening, maintenance, catering);
- staff sensitivity groups.

I will conclude with some consideration of the benefits and risks of groups in therapeutic communities. Groups provide the vehicle through which core aspects of the therapeutic community model are put into effect, including peer support and feedback, shared decision making, social learning and reality confrontation. The risks include the destructive use of peer pressure on individuals and a collusive denial of reality, in extreme cases leading to what Hobson has called the 'messianic' community.

The question 'How are groups used in therapeutic communities?' requires two different answers. On the one hand, a therapeutic community is itself a group-living situation. On the other hand, different kinds of groups are used within a therapeutic community.

# The therapeutic community as a group-living situation

A simple explanation of the theory of how a therapeutic community works is something like this. The community provides the opportunity for its members to interact as they do in their lives outside the community – at home, at work, in their personal relationships, etc. In fact, they cannot help behaving as they usually do because it is too difficult to keep up with a pretense for 24 hours a day. Sooner or later, maladaptive responses will become apparent (e.g., when they feel under pressure or are upset or angry). These responses provide the material that can then be discussed, explored and understood, with other members sharing their own experiences. Out of this process, suggestions arise for how to respond differently when a similar situation occurs, which the member can try to practise, the result in turn being available for discussion and learning, and so on in a repeated cycle along the lines of Kolb's experiential learning cycle (Kolb, 1984). These discussions often take place in the group meetings, but can also and importantly take place in informal times outside the main structure of the day.

## Historical context

Communities designed to provide shelter and care for people suffering from severe mental ill health have a long history: from Gheel in Belgium in the fourteenth century, to The Retreat in York in the late eighteenth and early nineteenth centuries, where the method known as 'moral treatment' was developed. What we now call 'therapeutic communities' emerged in the twentieth century, in which the aim was not only to provide shelter and care, but to use the environment as an opportunity for social engagement and learning – about oneself and others – in order to ameliorate as far as possible the individual's trouble in living.

Tom Main, who coined the term 'therapeutic community' while working at Northfield military psychiatric hospital during the Second World War, described it as:

> an attempt to use a hospital not as an organization run by doctors in the interests of their own greater technical efficiency, but as a community with the immediate aim of full participation of all its members in its daily life and the eventual aim of the resocialization of the neurotic individual for life in ordinary society.
>
> (Main, 1946)

Another useful definition was provided by Maxwell Jones, probably the best-known pioneer of the therapeutic community:

> What distinguishes a therapeutic community from other comparable treatment centres is the way in which the institution's total resources, staff, patients,

and their relatives, are self-consciously pooled in furthering treatment. That implies, above all, a change in the usual status of patients.

(Jones, 1968, pp. 85–86)

During the Second World War, the target population of therapeutic communities at Northfield Hospital, and at Mill Hill Hospital where Maxwell Jones was in charge, were soldiers that today would be diagnosed with PTSD or other stress-related disorders. After the War, therapeutic communities were introduced into a number of different settings. Probably the best known of these was Henderson Hospital, which specialised in the treatment of people with severe personality disorders (originally called 'psychopaths'), and where four practice principles were identified in research by the sociologist Rapoport (1960):

1   *Communalism:* There should be tight-knit intimate sets of relationships, with sharing of amenities (dining room, etc.), use of first names, and free communication.
2   *Permissiveness:* All members should tolerate from one another a wide degree of behaviour that might be distressing or seem deviant by ordinary standards.
3   *Democratisation:* Every member of the community should share equally in the exercise of power in decision making about community affairs.
4   *Reality confrontation:* Residents should be continuously presented with interpretations of their behaviour as it is seen by others, in order to counteract their tendency to distort, deny or withdraw from their difficulties in getting on with others.

Other settings developed and adapted these principles to meet the needs of different populations. These included large mental hospitals, day hospitals, prisons and secure units, schools for maladjusted children (where therapeutic community principles had been used since the beginning of twentieth century before the term was coined), and a range of independent organisations for people with learning disabilities or with acute or long-term mental health needs.

In this chapter, I will focus on three types of therapeutic community that were developed to meet the needs of individuals experiencing psychosis: psychiatric wards using a therapeutic community approach; 'alternative' asylum for people experiencing acute psychosis; and community-based settings for the rehabilitation/recovery of people with long-term psychosis.

## The therapeutic community approach

The 'therapeutic community approach' was the term used by David Clark to distinguish it from the 'therapeutic community proper' which followed the principles developed at Henderson Hospital for small specialised units for selected residents (Clark, 1965). In contrast, the therapeutic community approach was designed to meet the needs of patients and staff of large mental hospitals where inmates often showed the effects of institutionalisation. It was 'in some degree a revival of the principles of moral treatment' and emphasised 'open doors, full activity, increased freedom and responsibility' (Clark, 1965). In particular, the therapeutic community approach encouraged staff to see the patients as human beings worthy of respect and able to participate as far as possible in decisions about their own care and treatment. In a telling phrase, Clark said that he 'gave the nurses a chance to do for the patients the things they'd always wanted to'. In summary, the therapeutic community approach was intended to be a way of revitalising mental hospitals, tapping into latent reserves of idealism and humanity in the staff, and latent potential for social engagement in the patients. For further reading, see Mandelbrote (1965) and Clark (1996).

## Alternative asylum

Alternatives to hospital have been developed to provide a safe, containing place for people experiencing a sudden onset of psychosis or a relapse, but who do not want to be admitted to hospital. Many of these originated in what was known as the 'anti-psychiatry' movement, associated with the work of R.D. Laing and David Cooper. Laing founded the Philadelphia Association which established an alternative asylum at Kingsley Hall in 1965 (Berke, 1980). From this evolved networks of houses located in residential neighbourhoods which were characterised by the absence of any distinction between residents with professional qualifications and residents with severe mental health needs. Responsibility for day-to-day living and household chores was shared informally. Although this was group living, there were few formally structured group meetings: instead, the emphasis was on informal support in a low-stress environment, with either no or minimum use of medication. Contemporary examples of alternative asylum include the Arbours Association (Berke, Masoliver and Ryan, 1995), Soteria Houses (Ciompi and Hoffman, 2004), and various crisis houses run by statutory or independent organisations.

## Therapeutic communities in the community

Evolving out of the hospital-based therapeutic community approach on the one hand and alternatives to asylum on the other – both of which de-emphasised the distinction between the roles of 'patient' and 'staff', and promoted the therapeutic value of ordinary human interaction and everyday tasks – a number of projects have been developed to meet the needs of people with long-term severe mental health problems. These include communities in houses in residential urban areas, and ones in rural settings with an emphasis on engagement with nature – a movement that has become known as Green Care, which was the subject of a special issue of the journal *Therapeutic Communities* in 2008 (Sempik, 2008). Communities derive their theoretical perspectives from a variety of sources – for example, Heidegger (Gale, 2000) and Buddhism (Hickey, 2008) – but the implementation usually includes a daily community meeting and subgroups that meet as work groups or for group therapy.

## Different kinds of groups in therapeutic communities

Groups of various types form a central part of therapeutic community practice, providing opportunities for peer support and feedback, shared decision making, social learning and reality confrontation.

### Community meetings

The key activity of most therapeutic communities is the regular community meeting of all staff and patients/clients/residents,[1] usually held daily, but at least once a week. The main functions of the community meeting can be described as follows (Kennard, 1998):

- *To maximise the sharing of information.* Simply by being present, everyone is kept up-to-date with the life of the community. Anyone who has information to tell the rest of the community (whether reporting events or giving opinions) has an effective means of doing so. The community meeting is thus a kind of living newspaper of the community.
- *To build a sense of cohesion and belonging within the community.* Everyone can get to know the other members; they can participate, silently or vocally, in the sharing of their own and others' hopes and fears, problems and achievements, and this builds a sense of being part of a community.
- *To make open and public the process of decision making.* In some communities, residents and staff decide jointly what to do about a particular matter affecting one of them or the community as a whole. In other communities, certain decisions may be made by the leader of the community or by the staff together. In both situations, the way decisions are made is transparent. This contrasts with the 'Kafkaesque' quality of other institutions, where decisions are made in hidden places and are handed down in a way that makes the recipients feel helpless to do anything about it (a situation familiar to the staff and inmates of many traditional institutions).
- *To provide a forum for personal 'feedback'.* Group meetings provide a forum for people to give and receive personal reactions from one another, where participants learn how they are seen not just by one other person but by many, and where – depending on the feedback – they can try to be less aggressive, demanding or self-effacing; to listen more, to take more interest in others; or to enact whatever change is suggested. Group meetings also provide a vehicle for community members to exert pressure on an individual whose attitudes or behaviour is disturbing or upsetting to others, or threatens their own wellbeing. This goes one step further than simply giving feedback which the individual can choose to accept or ignore. The pressure might be in the form of an exhortation: 'Why don't you try asking more politely next time you want to

watch the other television channel?' or it can take the form of a verbal 'contract' to change a particular way of behaving.

These functions require the face-to-face contact in a large circle of all staff and patients. In communities for people with chronic psychosis, in particular for those who are socially withdrawn, some members may be unwilling to attend or may only attend for part of a meeting. There can be a difficult balance for staff to manage between respecting the patient's autonomy in not attending meetings and encouraging or persuading them to attend. Staff themselves may also find reasons not to attend – pressing matters to deal with or paperwork to complete. Issues of reluctance and ambivalence about attending meetings are to be expected, and need regular discussion if they are to be understood and challenged and not allowed to undermine the norms and culture of the therapeutic community.

### Small-group therapy

In addition to community meetings, in many therapeutic communities members are allocated to a small group that meets once, twice or three times a week. Each group (there may be two or three depending on the size of the community) has a consistent membership, with the same patients and staff meeting each time. The small group can provide a focus for attachment within the community and allows issues to be explored in more depth than is possible in the community meeting. Where the therapeutic community is operating as an admission ward or providing training placements for staff, there may be a fairly high turnover of group members.

---

### Clinical vignette 12.1

A man, who was initially invited into a small-group therapy session by a patient as a friend-cum-guardian, continued to attend the regular sessions in the absence of the patient. This man began to take a leading role in the group, asking questions in an insensitive way and intimidating the inexperienced therapists by claiming to have had training as a psychoanalyst. This was presented in supervision as a problem concerning how to cope with a difficult newcomer, and the supervisor had to point out that this man was not actually a member of the group and had no business there in the absence of the patient who had invited him.

*Comment:* The staff had become so used to the boundaries of membership being highly permeable that they had come to accept anyone who presented themselves as a member. Clarifying the existence of boundaries and categories of membership – however wide – enabled them to see that their task was not to cope with the interloper but to extrude him, which they did.

---

## Task groups

Task or work groups provide the opportunity for members to engage in meaningful practical tasks that make a contribution to the community and also provide a vehicle for social interaction. The nature of the work will depend on the capacities of the members and the resources of the therapeutic community. Communities in rural settings make a virtue of the opportunities for gardening. Other tasks may include cleaning, helping with administration, showing visitors around, organising an outing or helping in the kitchen. Whatever the task, the goal is therapeutic – to learn from the activity. For people suffering from chronic and severe mental illness, the capacity to engage in task groups will be limited and initially one-to-one support may be needed.

---

### Clinical vignette 12.2

In a therapeutic community for people with long-term severe mental illness, a decorating project was organised, to be carried out by the weekly maintenance group. We started to involve the clients gradually. First of all, we showed the clients what to do with the brushes and the paint. Then we did the physical work with them, and discussed the details of the painting task as it progressed. Once the first few clients had engaged, others came to join, having seen that it was okay and that others seemed to be enjoying it. We were able to break down the clients' initial questions, such as 'What is the point?' into smaller, more manageable questions such as, 'Shall I use this colour or that one?' and 'Where shall I begin to paint?' The actual doing of the task together in the group provided the beginning of a response to their initial question of 'What is the point?' Indeed, clients started to feel that they belonged and that their contribution made a difference. Some clients began to talk about how they would decorate their own flats when they moved on; others talked about decorating their room in the house; others about when to take a break and start work again; and so forth.

(*Source:* Handover, 2000)

---

## Creative arts therapy groups

Many therapeutic communities use creative therapy groups as part of the weekly programme. These provide an alternative, mainly nonverbal way, to explore members' feelings and experiences. Art therapy is the most commonly used modality, but others include music therapy, drama therapy and psychodrama. A full account of the group in art therapy is given in Chapter 20.

## Staff sensitivity groups

Staff sensitivity groups play a particularly important role in therapeutic communities, along with other regular staff groups such as the staff review meeting immediately following a community meeting. The relatively equal status of staff and patients, with the sharing of tasks and the culture of openness, mean that staff are exposed as real persons. They cannot hide behind formal job titles or in precisely defined roles. At the same time, they have a professional job to do: to facilitate patients' engagement with the therapeutic programme, to promote and manage group interaction, to monitor and, where helpful, to interpret behaviour and processes, especially if these threaten to undermine the smooth running of the community.

This combination of openness and exposure, along with maintaining a professional role, is a major challenge that requires frequent examination. A staff member may experience confusion over where to draw the line between a personal and professional relationship with a patient, or may be angry or upset over an incident that was not properly managed or contained, or may need support in a difficult ongoing situation. Tensions between staff can also arise and the dynamics of the staff team need constant monitoring so that hidden or latent conflicts can be brought into the open and discussed. If the staff cannot do this among themselves, they will be less able to do it for the community as a whole.

The weekly sensitivity group is like the lubricant that keeps the machine running, as also are the staff groups that meet to reflect after each community meeting. Without them, anxieties, tensions and conflicts can easily lead to a situation in which staff members become emotionally defensive and are unable to engage fully and openly in the life of the community.

## Benefits and risks of a therapeutic community

The benefits of a therapeutic community can be separated into its culture and its outcomes. The culture includes reducing the difference in status between staff and patients, involving the patient as an equal or near equal partner in responsibility for their own and others' therapy and for the running of the community, and using the everyday life of the community as the material for therapy. There are also benefits for staff training – learning what it is like to be a patient and how you appear to others when formal roles are not available.

The outcome benefits for people suffering from acute psychosis have been evaluated for the Soteria model. Two Soteria houses, in California and Berne, have been subjected to randomised or matched control trials to compare them with usual hospital treatment. In both studies, the 2-year outcomes were at least as good in the Soteria group, even though less antipsychotics were prescribed for the Soteria group (Ciompi and Hoffman, 2004). Evaluation of the outcome for people with long-term mental health needs has been largely qualitative, and is as much about changing the culture of the institution and the attitudes of staff as it is about changes for the patients (Campling, Davies and Farquharson, 2004).

The benefit for staff is reflected in the value placed on therapeutic community experience in training for mental health staff. Transient therapeutic communities have been attended by over 1,200 mental health professionals in a span of 20 years. A recent report on these concluded that therapeutic communities:

> [. . .] are effective learning and personal development tools; use powerful processes which have a positive impact on participants, and their awareness of their own and others' personal and interpersonal dynamics and behaviour; and produce effective interpersonal and enabling environments.
>
> (Lees, et al., 2016)

However, any powerful tool has risks – and therapeutic communities are no exception. Roberts (1980) has written about a number of potential destructive processes that can occur in therapeutic communities. These include destructive behaviour by an individual who is feeling alienated from the community, is unmotivated or has become overly dependent on the community, and destructive group phenomena including splitting and projection, subculturing and scapegoating. A common form of group splitting is when one group attributes its own negative or unwanted attributes to another group. For example, the staff group may disown their own propensity to sickness or irrationality and attribute this to the patient group, or attribute their own insensitive, autocratic tendencies to a higher management group. The dynamics in a therapeutic community are particularly well described by Tom Main (1975).

A risk that is inherent in the breaking down of barriers between staff and patient roles is that the relationship between a staff and patient member may become counter-therapeutic in some way. This may be in agreeing to keep secret information that ought to be communicated to the rest of the community, in developing an exclusive relationship that undermines involvement with the community as a whole, or in inappropriate physical intimacy. Such risks require sensitive monitoring and a culture of openness so that potential or actual breaches of the boundary between a professional and personal relationship – i.e., when the relationship threatens to undermine rather than facilitate therapy – can be openly discussed and lessons learned.

Finally, the attractiveness of the therapeutic community approach has inevitably led to attempts to introduce the model without a full understanding or commitment to making it work. Probably the best known example of tokenism is the fictional portrayal of a ward meeting in the film *One Flew Over the Cuckoo's Nest* (1975). Ward meetings may be set up with no clear idea of how they should run and no training, supervision or support for the staff with responsibility for running them. One study of a 450-bed hospital which had 220 groups meeting regularly found that the staff had a general lack of clarity about the groups' structure, purpose, functioning and theoretical framework, and that many groups 'served only to increase anxiety or to reflect the anxieties and defences of the units they served', although there were 'notable exceptions' (Robertson and Davison, 1997). A case example of a poorly understood ward meeting with commentaries by four experienced clinicians is provided in Bell and Novakovic (2013).

## Summary

Therapeutic communities have been called living–learning situations. The experience of living as a member of a community calls forth the members' problems (psychological, emotional and social) in events that parallel outside life. This occurs in such a way that they are: (1) visible to everyone; (2) available for discussion when other members can share similar experiences and offer feedback and suggestions; and (3) can be modified through practice. This cycle can be repeated as often as needed. Thus therapeutic communities operate as group-living situations, within which are a variety of specific groups. The core group is the community meeting, with smaller groups meeting for different specific purposes.

The therapeutic community can be seen as a modality, a framework, rather than one theoretical model. The format can be used with different theoretical lenses – psychoanalytic, systemic, group analytic, behavioural, spiritual and philosophical. These explanatory models help staff to make sense of their roles and can be used to guide staff–patient interactions and understanding. As a framework, the therapeutic community offers unique opportunities for therapeutic learning, for both staff and patients, as literally everything that happens is open to examination. Such a powerful tool is not without risks, and appropriate staff training and supervision are essential in order to avoid or manage these risks.

## Note

1    All three terms are in use depending on the setting. I will usually use the term 'patient', but will use them all interchangeably.

## References

Bell, D. and Novakovic, A. (2013) 'A community meeting on an acute psychiatric ward: Observation and commentaries' in *Living on the Border*. London: Karnac.

Berke, J.H. (1980) 'Therapeutic community models: II Kingsley Hall' in E. Jansen (Ed), *The Therapeutic Community*. London: Croom-Helm.

Berke, J.H., Masoliver, C. and Ryan, T.J. (1995) *Sanctuary: The Arbours experience of alternative community care*. London: Process Press.

Campling, P., Davies, S. and Farquharson, G. (2004) *From Toxic Institutions to Therapeutic Environments*. Gaskell: London.

Ciompi, L. and Hoffman, H. (2004) Soteria Berne: An innovative milieu therapeutic approach to acute schizophrenia based on the concept of affect-logic. *World Psychiatry*, 3(3), 140–146.

Clark, D.H. (1965) The therapeutic community – Concept, practice and future. *The British Journal of Psychiatry*, 131, 553–564.

Clark, D.H. (1996) *The Story of a Mental Hospital*. London: Process Press.

Gale, J. (2000) 'The dwelling place of meaning' in S. Tucker (Ed), *A Therapeutic Community Approach to Care in the Community.* London: Jessica Kingsley.

Handover, K. (2000) 'Building a home of one's own' in S Tucker (Ed), *A Therapeutic Community Approach to Care in the Community.* London: Jessica Kingsley.

Hickey, B. (2008) Lothlorien community: A holistic approach to recovery from mental health problems. *Therapeutic Communities, 29*(3), 261–272.

Jones, M. (1968) *Social Psychiatry in Practice.* Penguin: Harmondsworth.

Kennard, D. (1998) *An Introduction to Therapeutic Communities.* London: Jessica Kingsley.

Kolb, D.A. (1984) *Experiential Learning: Experience as the source of learning and development.* Englewood Cliffs, NJ: Prentice-Hall.

Lees, J., Haigh, R., Lombardo, A. and Rawlings, B. (2016) Transient therapeutic communities: The 'living-learning experience' trainings. *Therapeutic Communities, 37*(2), 57–68.

Main, T. (1946) The hospital as a therapeutic institution. *Bulletin of the Menninger Clinic,* 10, 66–70.

Main, T. (1975) 'Some psychodynamics of large groups' in L. Kreeger (Ed), *The Large Group.* London: Constable.

Mandelbrote, B.M. (1965) The use of psychodynamic and sociodynamic principles in the treatment of psychotics. *Comprehensive Psychiatry, 6*(6), 381–387.

Rapoport, R.N. (1960) *Community as Doctor.* London: Tavistock.

Roberts, J.P. (1980) Destructive processes in a therapeutic community. *International Journal of Therapeutic Communities, 1*(3), 159–170.

Robertson, S. and Davison, S. (1997) A survey of groups within a psychiatric hospital. *Psychoanalytic Psychotherapy,* 11, 119–133.

Sempik, J. (2008) Green Care: A natural resource for therapeutic communities? [Editorial]. *Therapeutic Communities, 29*(3), 221–227.

# Chapter 13

# The development and some specific features of group psychotherapeutic treatment in forensic units

*Tija Žarković Palijan, Ana Magerle,*
*Sonja Petković, Editha Vučić*

## Introduction

Forensic psychotherapy, as well as forensic psychiatry in general, is a relatively young discipline that is still evolving, but the interest in this field has grown in the last few decades. In general, the meaning of the term 'forensic psychotherapy' involves the application of psychological therapies in the treatment of crime offenders suffering from mental disorders (McGauley and Humphrey, 2003). However, it is fair to say that the context of forensic psychiatry is dominated by the psychodynamic method (Welldon, 1994), since the very development of this discipline is based on a psychoanalytic viewpoint.

One of the main functions of forensic psychotherapy emphasises the use of psychodynamic principles in understanding unconscious impulses and fantasies, and how they are reflected in the behaviour and interactions of the patient. McGauley (2002) points out that, despite the theories that forensic patients cannot understand the psychodynamic process, forensic psychotherapy in closed institutions encompasses much more than individual treatment. Since the essence of psychotherapy is in gaining control (Xenitidis, Barnes and White, 2005), there is mistrust of psychotherapy used within the forensic psychiatric field. However, it is reported in literature that the application of the psychodynamic concept can help in understanding the phenomenology, even in psychotic patients (McGauley, 2002). Group analysis, as well as any analytical psychotherapy, is more an emotional than intellectual experience (Hoffmann and Kluttig, 2006). In fact, experience and research from the Portman Clinic prove that for most patients, group psychotherapy is an excellent choice (Woods and Williams, 2014).

Forensic psychiatric patients are often people who, as a result of abuse and/or neglect in childhood, have developed numerous, severe and chronic mental disorders. The task of a forensic psychotherapist is to evaluate and treat the patients, consult with colleagues, supervise younger colleagues and professional teams, and give support to the staff in a forensic institution. Furthermore, they carry out the assessment of psychopathology and the assessment of risk and of various capabilities for the purposes of the criminal court (Adshead, 2001).

## Forensic psychotherapy treatment

Forensic psychotherapy involves four basic types of activities: direct clinical work (assessment and treatment), supervision, clinical meetings, and consultations or institutional supervision. It is the work of a whole team that, in addition to medical staff, includes clinical psychologists, psychotherapists, social workers, social pedagogues, special education teachers, occupational therapists and experts of other related professions who are trained to work with specific populations (Cordess and Cox, 1996).

Traditionally, psychoanalysis used to imply above-average intelligence as a prerequisite for the patient to be involved, or even to be referred to psychotherapy. However, contemporary psychodynamic psychotherapy has evolved over the years by expanding the theory and practice, and today includes (either in experimental or the applied clinical sense) populations that were once considered unsuitable, for example, people with psychosis, severe mental disease, or the elderly (Xenitidis, Barnes and White, 2005).

Treatment can be individual, group or within a therapeutic community (McGauley and Humphrey, 2003). It can take place in therapeutic programmes in the community or as a hospital outpatient, and provides a variety of treatment models. The nature of the environment in which the treatment takes place largely determines the goals and course of treatment. The Portman Clinic applies psychoanalytic group therapy in the treatment process of the most severe and difficult patients (Woods and Williams, 2014).

In addition to providing treatment within a closed forensic psychiatric institution, the task of the expert team is also to assess the psychological progress and possibilities of transfer to lower-security wards. However, safety issues and risks are more pronounced in a closed institution, so the experts often face a conflict of roles: that of the therapist and of the assessor (McGauley and Humphrey, 2003). That is to say, the conflict is between responsibility to the patient and responsibility to society (Magerle, 2001). The issue of setting up security within the institution often overshadows the need for treatment and undermines the implementation of therapeutic activities. Therefore, the expert team must work towards achieving a balance in control, care and treatment (Norton and McGauley, 2000). It is therefore necessary to encourage the development of specialised methods and disciplines for use in a forensic psychiatric context.

The most commonly applied approach in psychiatry in general, and thus also in forensic psychiatry, is the psychodynamic approach to treatment. Hence therapy work in groups is becoming increasingly preferred. Before and during treatment, the forensic psychotherapist should take into account the context in which the treatment takes place. If she/he estimates that the overall situation is unsatisfactory, then supportive therapy is at first more necessary than therapy focused on self-analysis. The period of supportive therapy can then pave the way for a more active treatment; for example, individual psychodynamic therapy or group psychotherapy (Norton and McGauley, 2000). In *Cognitive Analytic Therapy for Offenders,*

Pollock and colleagues (2006) present cognitive analytic therapy as a new form of forensic psychotherapy, which may include understanding, conceptualisation, treatment and management in dealing with crime offenders.

Many psychiatric patients need permanent or at least frequent communication with the therapist. In recent times, there has been consideration of the application of telemedicine, specifically telepsychiatry, in achieving the best possible results. Telemedicine, thanks to the expansion of communication technologies, provides medical services from a distance (McLaren, 2003). Although this method is very new and needs further research, many authors already emphasise positive results, especially as relates to the cost benefit.

## Supervision in forensic psychotherapy

According to Cox (1996), supervision is indispensable: *conditio sine qua non*. It is an essential tool in the development of a number of professions, including psychotherapy (Cottrell, 1999). Therapists have supervision on an individual and group level (Klain, 2007), and it can be in informal or more structured conditions (i.e., on the wards or during the presentation of a case). A group supervision can include several individual therapists who together discuss individual sessions, but it can also refer to group therapy (Cox, 1996). For example, Klain (2007) writes about the supervision of a group therapy for psychotic patients. The objectives of institutional supervision include the understanding of how psychopathology of patients can be identified, investigated, and incorporated into certain aspects of the functioning of the institution.

## The authors' own experience and research

In the Dr. Ivan Barbot neuropsychiatric hospital in Popovača, the department of forensic psychiatry, with a total of 200 beds, has the largest capacity for the treatment of mentally incompetent persons, or for the enforcement of involuntary confinement under the Law on the Protection of Persons with Mental Disabilities, in Croatia. At the end of the 1970s, Klain began training doctors and nurses in the hospital, and he introduced group psychotherapy as a treatment method for psychotic patients. We were the first department in Croatia to use psychodynamic groups in the treatment of psychotic forensic psychiatric patients, and this training is still ongoing.

Each department in the hospital is run as a separate sociotherapeutic community, offering individual, group and family psychotherapy, along with sociotherapy in the strict sense and through occupational activities. Composed of mixed diagnostic groups, the community is modified according to the needs and functioning of the patients. Hence a group may include patients with mental retardation, chronic psychotic patients, patients with alcohol issues, and forensic psychiatric patients on parole who attend as outpatients. Besides being treated in the sociotherapeutic community of the forensic psychiatric department, alcoholics are

also referred to the day programme of the sociotherapeutic community of alcoholics in the hospital. Other diagnostic groups, mainly from the psychosis group,
participate in other sociotherapeutic groups and group sessions of psychodynamic
orientation.

Across the sociotherapeutic communities, patients form groups of 8 to 10
members, in order to take part in occupational activities once a week. Lasting
60 minutes, the groups are analytically oriented, and work on the 'door ajar'
principle. Each group includes an observer and a supervisor – after each session,
the supervisor conducts an interview with the therapist and the observer. Finally,
there is an overall supervision with all the therapists and observers involved in
group psychotherapy in the hospital.

### Research into group dynamics in forensic psychotherapy

Although forensic psychiatric patients formally agree to group therapy, the treatment is compulsory. Thus, patients consider the therapists and the environment
to be the extended arm of the authorities, i.e., the criminal court. In this way, the
department is a prison, the medical staff are prison guards, the group is a courtroom,
and the therapist is an investigator or a judge. This view is corroborated by the fact
that the doctor–therapist is the person who proposes to the court the termination
of forced confinement. Forensic psychiatric patients, whose goal is to get out of
the hospital/confinement as quickly as possible, often believe that they may be
dismissed if they behave well, and not because their health has improved. Patients
hence find the process of transition of group dynamics from the initial to the
so-called intermediate stage to be time consuming and onerous. This involves a
transition from monologue and to dialogue, with an emphasis on the here-and-now
and a requirement to discuss the taboo topic (i.e., the offence).

In order to expedite the transition process, that is, to eliminate the factor
(doctor–therapist) that we thought was slowing it down, we agreed with the
supervisor to let the therapists form groups in departments in which they did not
work. In this way, we wanted to achieve a faster coherence of the group. However,
after a year of work with groups in other departments, we noticed that the problem
had not changed. We assumed the reason for this was the impact of a large group
(i.e., the department) on the dynamics of a small group (i.e., the therapy group);
departments vary in education and approach to the patient, as well as a difference
in departmental atmosphere.

We conducted a study in which we were monitoring the development of group
dynamics in two groups of patients: Group A from Department 1 and Group B
from Department 2, with the same therapist and observer. Each group had
10 members (eight patients, a therapist and an observer), working on the 'door
ajar' principle. The patients were schizophrenic, and occasionally there was a
patient from another psychiatric category in the group. All patients had committed
murder or attempted murder. The average age of patients in Group A was 33 years,
and in Group B was 34 years; the average duration of hospitalisation in Group

A was 29.6 months, while in Group B it was 30.3 months; there were no other statistically significant differences.

The following is a summary of our findings, after observing the events and the dynamics of group cohesion over a year:

- Group A very soon overcomes the so-called initial phase, while Group B is, after a year of work, practically still in the first stage. When an acute psychotic patient is discovered to be in the groups, it does not increase anxiety in Group A as the group assumes the role of a therapist and confronts the patient with the disease. Yet Group B rejects the psychotic patient due to growing anxiety in the group. In a similar vein, when a new member is introduced into the groups, Group A is friendly, and helps the new member to adapt to the new situation. In Month 11 of group work, two members of Group A suggest to the other group members that they include a patient who is doing very badly (and has repeatedly attempted suicide): members of the group think the group could help him, as it has helped them. Meanwhile in Group B, having released one patient, the therapist raises the question of introducing a new patient to the group. The group is silent, and after the therapist repeats the question, one member says: 'They could bring in all new members because we have been in the group for a long time.'

- Group A very quickly establishes trust between group members. In the intermediate stage, with occasional excursions into the final stage, Group A openly discusses the perpetrated offences, with communication directed towards all members of the group. When a group member leaves the group because he is released from hospital, Group A reacts with pleasure. They see the release of the patient as a success for the whole group, who have helped in his treatment. It is also the proof that all members may soon go home, too. However, Group B is angry because they think that the group member has not deserved the release and that he will not be able to manage at home.

- When the therapist is absent in the initial group meetings, Groups A and B have the same reaction: they express satisfaction when the group is cancelled. However, in Month 12, even though they have been told that the group is cancelled, Group A still gather at their regular time because they have seen the therapist at the hospital. (The therapist is in fact on holiday and is at the hospital for some other reason.) In contrast, Group B has the same satisfied reaction as they did in the beginning of the group work when they hear of the cancellation.

- In both groups, technical issues are discussed in almost every session. For example: who is in charge of releasing a patient, what kind of medical treatment they receive, various issues related to leave, etc.

- Some behaviour is only observed in Group B: patients are regularly late for meetings; the place for the session is often not prepared; the staff persistently call out the patients for the session; and patients are often sent for tests during the session or have other obligations (for example, an occupational therapist telephones the group therapist to ask him to release a patient from participation in the group).

After a year of work in groups and monitoring the group processes, we interviewed the staff of both departments about their views on a variety of therapeutic procedures. We discovered that personnel in Department 1 had received training in psychodynamics, as well as other forms of therapy in psychiatry. Every afternoon, when there was no doctor in the department, Department 1 personnel would lead meetings of large groups. Most of them also lead small therapy groups.

We then conducted a survey of staff at every department. In an anonymous survey, the staff were asked to rate every therapy procedures (pharmacological, occupational, sociotherapeutic community, and individual and group psychotherapy) on a scale of 1 (lowest) to 5 (highest). According to the results, there were no statistically significant differences in the attitudes of personnel in Departments 1 and 2 to pharmacological therapy, occupational therapy, sociotherapeutic community and individual psychotherapy. However, a statistically significant difference ($t = 2.89$) was found in the rate of group psychotherapy: the staff of Department 1 gave group psychotherapy an average grade of 4.20, and the staff of Department 2 gave grade 3.21 (Magerle, 2001).

Based on the research, we concluded that the overall atmosphere in the department has a huge impact on the development and success of group therapy, in particular in forensic psychiatric departments. This implies a certain level of staff training, positive attitude towards therapeutic technique or method, own experience, positive attitude towards the patient, understanding of their offences, and above all, a common motivation towards changing our attitudes in dealing with such patients (Balint groups). According to our research and our later psychotherapeutic experience and monitoring, we can conclude that in the first stage, as well as in all other stages of the group process development, the relationships in the larger group (the department) are reflected in its smaller part (the therapy group). Depending on their quality, they can motivate or obstruct the group process development. The therapist's task is to identify this and to adapt his/her interventions with maximum patience. Iatrogenic effects within the group also have certain positive and negative impacts on the larger whole (the department).

After a certain time, the patients in these groups feel chosen, as having a special status, which sometimes leads to acting out. Here it is necessary to point out that in the beginning of the group work, we see the reverse effect, as the patients often wonder why it is that they are chosen, with negative and suspicious connotations. In the beginning of work with the groups, the patients did not allow the recording of the session (partly due to paranoia, and partly a lack of experience with trials).

This study has further strengthened our view that the therapist in a psychosis group can also be department doctor. We believe that in working with forensic psychiatric and homicidal patients, in these conditions, it is desirable that the same therapist heals both the body and the soul. Hence the therapist can be recognised as a good and bad object.

## Experience of group dynamics in forensic psychotherapy

In forensic psychiatric patients, we encounter destruction that has passed from words to action. Most of them have expressed the destruction in the harshest way possible – murder. Destruction is a way of communication, and communication in psychotic patients is blocked in two directions: blockage of their own communication (understanding their own needs), and blockage of communication with others. In a group with homicidal psychotic patients, the therapist is trying to establish communication with the destructive part and make it recognisable and comprehensible to the patient, because a therapeutic group can withstand destructive aggression better than one-to-one analytical situations (Magerle, 2001). At the beginning of group work, the communication is directed towards the therapist, who in these conditions is also the treating physician. Forensic psychiatric patients expect the therapist to give them a task and a topic to talk about. At first, these are monologues or questions addressed to the therapist on medical therapy, going out, weekends, therapeutic leave, etc. The group only acts as a group when they are talking about different situations in the department, i.e., when they bring the large group into the small one. Such dynamics initially slow down the development of the group process, but the therapists should not be discouraged. With the help of the supervisor, they can continue to work with the forensic psychiatric patients, but they also need to complete their own staff training, both those with higher and secondary medical education, so that almost all staff have completed training in group therapy through Balint groups and their own experience in the group (Kovač, 2007).

The feelings of helplessness, inability and incompetence when dealing with these patients is a very difficult experience, which lessens with training and supervision, and even results in a more optimistic attitude towards psychotherapy. Working with trained nurses and technicians improves the lives of the patients in the ward, and group psychotherapy becomes more common (Klain, 2007). Group psychotherapy is indicated for patients with a weak ego, and forensic psychiatric patients' ego is the weakest. Group psychotherapy, next to other forms of treatment, is the method of choice for working with forensic patients. However, therapists who are studying other types of psychotherapeutic methods will certainly bring new developments in the future.

During the Croatian War of Independence, when there was a lack of medication, we observed a significant increase in the deterioration of basic disease. The number of deteriorations in patients in forensic departments who concurrently had group treatment was significantly lower than in patients who were not included in group psychotherapy treatment. Also, in patients who received group psychotherapy, despite the deterioration of the disease, we did not observe outbursts of aggression. In other patients, the deterioration of the disease was accompanied by aggressive–destructive outbursts that had been described at the commission of the crime.

A supervisor, after 30 years of work with groups of psychotic forensic patients, stated that group work helps therapists to help their seriously ill patients, for whom they often feel very negative emotions and who are the cause of their extreme frustration. Although fearing that his results are not adequate, the supervisor is convinced that group psychotherapy has helped psychotic forensic patients, and so research must be continued and developed further (Klain, 2007).

## Conclusion

Forensic psychotherapy, although a young discipline within psychiatry, includes a series of tasks and responsibilities. The quality of the treatment depends upon the proper selection and training of professionals who work with forensic psychiatric patients. Experts in mental health can and should use all methods and approaches that contribute to the understanding and wellbeing of the patient, but any action must be structured and planned by the whole professional team.

Some argue that dealing with forensic psychotherapy is not a prominent activity within professional psychotherapy, and, moreover, that it is depressing and frightening. Also, some experts cannot act in accordance with the fact that the care is more important than the cure. On the other hand, supporters of forensic psychotherapy emphasise that its goal is to reduce the suffering of the patient and that the provision of care is sometimes more challenging than the cure, and these are the facts that make the job both intellectually and humanistically delightful. Moreover, professionals who help people who are hopeless and helpless point out that it provides immense pleasure.

However, it should be noted that patients placed in high-risk institutions have a whole spectrum of chronic disorders. It is not always easy to communicate with people who have committed crimes because their interpersonal skills are often poor or completely lacking. Patients with complex psychopathology are often additionally burdened with various comorbidities that even further complicate the possibility of recovery. Therefore, an expert who decides to work with forensic patients should be prepared to deal with frustrations, accusations, fear, violence and responsibility on the one hand, and to maintain warmth, empathy, hope, faith and love on the other. It is crucial to stay balanced and to maintain objectivity.

## References

Adshead, G. (2001) Forensic psychotherapy. *BMJ Career Focus,* 323, S2-7316.

Cordess, C. and Cox, M. (1996) *Forensic Psychotherapy: Crime, psychodynamics and the offender patient.* London: Jessica Kingsley.

Cottrell, D. (1999) Supervision. *Advances in Psychiatric Treatment,* 5, 83–88.

Cox, M. (1996) 'A supervisor's view' (pp. 199–223) in C. Cordess and M. Cox (Eds), *Forensic Psychotherapy: Crime, psychodynamics and the offender patient.* London: Jessica Kingsley.

Hoffmann, K. and Kluttig, T. (2006) Psychoanalytic and group-analytic perspectives in forensic psychotherapy. *The Group-Analytic Society,* 39(1), 9–23.

Klain, E. (2007) 'Supervizija grupne psihoterapije sa psihotičnim forenzičnim pacijentima' (pp. 394–402) ['Supervision of group psychotherapy with psychotic forensic patients'] in T. Žarković Palijan and D. Kovačević (Eds), *Iz forenzične psihijatrije 2* [*From Forensic Psychiatry 2*]. Zagreb: Naklada Ceres.

Kovač, M. (2007) 'Dobit za bolnicu od edukacije iz grupne psihoterapije medicinskih sestara/tehničara' ['Benefits for the hospital from the group psychotherapy of psychiatric nurses'] in E. Klain and R. Gregurek (Eds), *Grupna psihoterapija* [*Group Psychotherapy*]. Zagreb: Medicinska naklada.

Magerle, A. (2001) 'Razvitak i neke specifičnosti grupno psihoterapijskog tretmana na forenzičkim odjelima' (pp. 355–362) ['Development and some specific features of group psychotherapeutic treatment in forensic departments'] in T. Žarković Palijan and D. Kovačević (Eds), *Iz forenzičke psihijatrije* [*From Forensic Psychiatry*]. Zagreb: Naklada Ceres.

McGauley, G. (2002) Forensic psychotherapy in secure settings. *The Journal of Forensic Psychiatry,* 13(1), 9–13.

McGauley, G. and Humphrey, M. (2003) Contribution of forensic psychotherapy to the care of forensic patients. *Advances in Psychiatric Treatment,* 9, 117–124.

McLaren, P. (2003) Telemedicine and telecare: What can it offer to mental health services? *Advances in Psychiatric Treatment,* 9, 54–61.

Norton, K. and McGauley, G. (2000) Forensic psychotherapy in Britain: Its role in assessment, treatment and training. *Criminal Behaviour and Mental Health,* 10, 82–90.

Pollock, P.H., Stowell-Smith, M. and Göpfert, M. (2006) *Cognitive Analytic Therapy for Offenders: A new approach to forensic psychotherapy.* London: Routledge.

Welldon, E. (1994) 'Forensic psychotherapy' (pp. 470–493) in P. Clarkson and M. Pokorny (Eds), *The Handbook of Psychotherapy.* London: Routledge.

Woods, J. and Williams, A. (2014) *Forensic Group Psychotherapy (The Portman Clinic Approach).* London: Karnac Books.

Xenitidis, K.I., Barnes, J. and White, J. (2005) Forensic psychotherapy for adults with learning disabilities: An inpatient group-analytic group. *Group Analysis,* 38(3), 427–438.

# Chapter 14

# Groups in early intervention services

## Group psychotherapy for patients with psychotic disorders in an early intervention programme (RIPEPP)

*Branka Restek-Petrović, Majda Grah,*
*Anamarija Bogović Dijaković, Nina Mayer*

## Introduction

The Early Intervention Programme for Psychotic Patients (RIPEPP) has existed at Sveti Ivan psychiatric hospital in Zagreb since 2005. It was designed and financed with hospital resources, and is based on: the psychodynamic theoretical framework of understanding psychotic disorders; years of experience in the application of modified group analysis in treating psychotic disorders; international experience in the application of group techniques in early intervention programmes; and experience with early intervention programmes in general (Addington and Addington, 2001; Woodhead, 2008).

Psychodynamic group psychotherapy of psychotic patients has been administered at Sveti Ivan hospital since 1990, and today it is a generally accepted therapeutic method in the clinical and outpatient treatment of psychotic and other psychiatric patients. In cooperation with the Zagreb Institute for Group Analysis and the Zagreb Medical School's Clinic for Psychological Medicine, the hospital has systematically encouraged and carried out the education of psychiatrists and other experts in various psychotherapeutic techniques, especially in group analysis, family therapy, psychoanalytic psychotherapy, cognitive behavioural therapy, and psychosocial methods of treatment.

## The RIPEPP programme

The RIPEPP programme involves patients at Sveti Ivan hospital receiving either inpatient or outpatient treatment who are in the 'critical period' of their psychotic disorders, within 5 years of the appearance of their first symptoms (Birchwood and Fiorillo, 2000). The RIPEPP programme is intended for patients with acute psychotic disorder, schizophrenia, schizoaffective disorder, delusional disorder, or bipolar affective disorder with psychosis, and it includes both patients and their family members.

The goal of the programme is the complete clinical and social recovery of the patient through the attainment of insight into the disorder and the acceptance of treatment, as well as the prevention of relapse. Psychodynamically speaking, the programme is intended to promote the creation of higher levels of object relations, a more cohesive self, and more mature defence mechanisms. The goals also include the adequate education of patients and their families as to the causes, onset, clinical presentation, and treatment of their disorder, as well as insight into early signs of the disorder. It also aims to correct maladaptive forms of behaviour, communication, and interpersonal relations within the family that may have a negative impact on maintaining remission. The programme consists of group psychotherapy and psychoeducation, psychosocial methods of treatment, and psychopharmacological therapy.

## Psychodynamic group psychotherapy

The therapeutic team of group analysts in the RIPEPP programme generally accept that group psychotherapy combined with antipsychotics is an effective method of treating psychotic disorders (Kanas, 1996; Gonzáles de Chávez, 2009). Led by a skilled therapist, we hold that a group of psychotic patients are, in the long term, capable of developing a group matrix (Foulkes, 1977), achieving significant communication and interaction, mutually supporting each other, using mirroring mechanisms, and introjecting some of the functions of the leader such that the group can become a therapeutic factor (Urlić, 1999).

The goals and therapeutic techniques in groups of psychotic patients generally differ depending on the theoretical approach of the therapist. Group analysts in our therapeutic team accept the conceptual position that psychotic disorders are a continuum of mental disorders, among which the psychoses are the most severe (Schermer and Pines, 1999; Urlić, 1999). Treatment is therefore optimistically oriented towards the possibility of attainment of higher levels of object relations, intersubjectivity and empathy. The function of group psychotherapy is not only to offer relief, support and elements of education, but also to enable internal changes. Patient groups are not designed to be solely places for 'adaptation training'; i.e., for the construction of a more functional and adaptable false self that is better suited to community norms (Schermer and Pines, 1999; Winnicott, 1965). Group therapy is also a place where the psychotic experience is transformed, where early traumatic experiences and primitive fantasies are discovered and analysed, and where psychological defence mechanisms are developed, leading to integral clinical and social recovery (Restek-Petrović, 2008).

Work with groups of young psychotic patients has led to insight into some specificities of the group process: reactions of sadness as a result of insight into the illness and its consequences, which brings the danger of suicide attempts; the need to analyse the traumatic experiences of psychotic episodes and hospitalisation, as well as the experience of psychopharmacological therapy; and the necessary integration of the psychotic experience into the personality. In terms of technique, experience has underlined the requirement for greater flexibility in boundaries: patients often leave the group due to a need for more independent functioning, but return when faced with a new psychotic episode. Experimenting with relationships in the group (friendships, romantic relationships) threaten the boundaries and integrity of the group. A wide range of technique is also needed; e.g., the use of humour, the acceptance of slang and youthful modes of expression, etc. (Restek-Petrović, et al., 2008, 2014).

### Inpatient group psychotherapy

The psychotherapy ward (where group psychotherapy begins as a part of the RIPEPP programme, after pharmacological intervention in the emergency ward) has 30 beds, and it is organised as a therapeutic community. The entire staff is trained in psychotherapy in the psychodynamic theoretical framework, and all employees have completed training as group analysts, group therapists or cognitive behavioural therapists. The therapy programme includes psychodynamic group psychotherapy four times per week. A one-hour median group session is run once a week by a psychiatrist–group analyst, while one-hour small group sessions are run three times a week by a group therapist nurse. The groups are divided into higher and lower levels based upon the maturity of their object relations, defence mechanisms and communications abilities (Yalom and Leszcz, 2005). Cognitive behavioural therapy workshops and psychoeducation are also part of the programme.

The ward staff attempts to create an atmosphere of safety, support and empathic acceptance within which the psychotherapy process begins. Work is performed on initial insight into the nature of the disorder, as well as into triggers that led to mental decompensation. A therapeutic alliance is forged with patients and their families, and patients are motivated to join the long-term, outpatient part of the RIPEPP programme.

## Clinical vignette 14.1

The first comment of the group is a patient: 'I can say that I had a nice weekend. I watched the match. I like football.' Another patient joins in that she also had a good weekend in the hospital, especially at the group sessions. After a short pause, Patient M speaks up, saying that she does not feel good because the devil is constantly following her, and that she managed to oppose him by watching a mass on television. She cannot go to church because she is to blame for her fiancé being in the locked ward because he was late to return. Patient V comments: 'One of the reasons I ended up here is because the devil or someone of his is following me, and then I get afraid, I start to shake. Since I've been here, I don't get afraid that often.' Patient L tries to comfort Patient M, saying that she is too self-critical, that she is always looking for something bad in herself, and that she is not to blame for her fiancé. Another patient asks Patient M: 'What does your devil look like?' Patient M says that she can feel him (she points over her shoulder) and that he is standing by her. Another patient points out that it is difficult to convince someone that these are psychotic symptoms, and that it is easier for Patient M to ascribe all her bad urges and negative feelings to someone else, for example the devil, than to herself. Patient L says that, before being hospitalised, he felt like a box full of Lego that he would always try to put together, but that someone else would always come and kick. While receiving treatment, he has realised that he can take the Lego out of the box and put them together into some shape.

*Comment:* Talk about symptoms is often a spontaneous subject in the group, and members of the group that are closer to recovery offer support, confrontation and reality testing to more acute patients.

## Clinical vignette 14.2

The first to contribute to the group is Patient T, who says how happy he is to be leaving the hospital soon. After him, Patient E and another patient also state their desire for the weekend to come as soon as possible so that they can go home too.

THERAPIST: Our thoughts are outside of the hospital, but how do we feel here in the group?
*A short silence ensues.*
PATIENT D: I've had enough of this hospital already, I'm sick of it all. I've been here for 3 months already. I was in the locked ward for a long time.
*Everyone laughs.*
PATIENT M: Man, you weren't well, what you did there was terrible.
PATIENT D *(laughing):* Yes, I insulted all of them, yelled at the doctors. You just have to relax a bit.
*Laughter.*
THERAPIST: Is it easier to discuss this kind of experience through a joke?

Patient T states how the horrible experience of the locked ward is behind them, but that he sees now that it was necessary after all. Patient D asks how the doctors know what is happening with them when they do not talk to them every day. Patient M points out that the groups are also important, that the staff observes them, but that they also signed consent to treatment themselves. The ward is open and they can leave when they want.

PATIENT E:  It's better for us to decide that together with the doctor.
PATIENT M:  But you ran away.
PATIENT E:  I didn't run away, I just had to take care of something.
PATIENT M:  But you had consequences.
PATIENT E:  I didn't: a few faxes were exchanged and that was all.
THERAPIST:  What does the group say about this: is it better to stay or to go?
PATIENT V:  I think you need to think about it: it's easy to leave, but you need to think about what the consequences might be.

The group advises Patient E to think it over, that she is going to leave the hospital anyway, and that everyone sees that she is getting better every day.

*Comment:* The experience and acceptance of treatment, and verbalisation of ambivalent transference towards the hospital and the staff, are frequent topics for discussion.

### Outpatient group psychotherapy

The outpatient RIPEPP programme includes long-term group psychodynamic psychotherapy for patients, group psychotherapy for their family members, and psychoeducational workshops for both groups together. Patients who lack the motivation or capacity for this type of psychotherapy are referred to psychosocial activities in the Patients' Club.

The perspective of a long-term group process offers the ability to work on self-consolidation and defence mechanisms, in order to develop object relations and to improve socialisation. After the analysis of the traumatic experience of their hospitalisation and their psychotic episode, and after establishing some insight into their disorder, patients with lower capacities and motivation leave the group, while some patients remain in treatment for years, with demanding therapeutic goals. One characteristic of early group work is the heightened activity of the therapist, who: incites communication and interaction; shows a supportive attitude; avoids interpreting subconscious content (especially in the early stages of group work); offers 'upward interpretations' when needed; and directs discussion more towards the 'here-and-now' rather than the 'there-and-then' (Restek-Petrović, 2004; Restek-Petrović, et al., 2016). After establishing cohesion and a group matrix, the therapist becomes less active and supportive, and can withdraw into the background. Yet the possibility of applying all kinds of therapeutic interventions remains because spontaneous communication and interaction create opportunities for the actualisation of internal conflicts in the group members.

After 11 years of the programme, nine psychotherapy groups are operating in the hospital today: eight groups with young psychotic patients and one group with older patients (in their 30s and 40s) who have experienced their first psychotic episode. The groups function on an 'open-door' principle, and patients remain in the group as long as necessary. After leaving a group, patients can continue treatment in the group if they have a relapse or if they need to work on new problems, as long as there is room for them in the group.

---

### Clinical vignette 14.3

Patient I begins the group session by boasting that her young daughter was praised at school, and so she let her play at a friend's house, despite her mother's disapproval. Patient E notes that Patient I has become more decisive in raising her daughter and no longer depends so much on her mother and her opinions. Patient I confirms this, and says that she met another mother at the school, that they had a nice conversation, and went for coffee together after the parent meeting.

Patient E continues by saying that, now that he has passed his last exam, he is beginning to think more and more about work, and that he imagines himself in the role of a professor, which is beginning to appeal to him more and more. He then looks at his 'modern' ripped jeans and wonders aloud how modern he can be dressed without risking his authority as a professor, while still remaining close to his students.

Patient L pensively comments that she has never really liked children, and could not imagine herself as a mother; but that when she sees how sweet and well behaved Patient I's daughter is, she thinks she might be able to be a mother someday too. Patient T, who graduated last summer, has been on a trip abroad with his family. He describes his new experience of security and satisfaction: he did not think of his illness, he took his medication, and enjoyed all the wonderful experiences.

Patient H joins in with the general good feeling: he was alone for a few days as his mother went on a trip. So he cooked for himself and he felt good. When she used to go away, he was anxious, he would constantly call and bother his brother or his uncle, and he would occasionally skip his medication. However, he now felt good to be alone.

The therapist comments that the whole group has grown up. Patient I is more sure in her role as a mother; Patient E is ready to embrace his professional role; Patient L is beginning to consider some new roles in life; Patient T is more relaxed outside the security of his home; and Patient H is enjoying the freedom of being alone. The group silently confirms this thought, and then Patient E states: 'It all somehow came about itself . . .'

*Comment:* All members of the group have been participating in the group for 5 or more years: one of the three university students has graduated while another has passed his last exam. In the past 2 years, the group members have gradually begun to associate with each other less frequently outside of the group sessions. In addition, other interactions outside the group are becoming more and more intense – looking for partners and new friends, trying new activities, enjoying time with their families and other joys in life, and the capacity to bear solitude.

## Clinical vignette 14.4

Patient C, a university student in her early 20s, is hospitalised for the first time due to a psychotic episode. She has difficulty with hospitalisation; she is untrusting and frightened. In the group sessions in the ward she is quiet, verbalising her fear of stigmatisation. At the suggestion of the therapist and her parents, she agrees to join the outpatient group.

At her first session, she sits in her coat, squeezing her bag in her lap. She introduces herself sparingly, accenting her student status and barely mentioning her illness. The mature group with a well-developed matrix acts supportively: the members encourage her to talk about her tests at university and her difficulties concentrating, while the other students in the group offer their own experiences. Patient C becomes more relaxed: after the group session, she goes for coffee with the other members.

*Comment:* Throughout the following 6 months, the establishment of a sealing-over mechanism is apparent, as is the stabilisation of the patient's condition and her advancement in socialisation. The experience of group cohesion and good symbiosis allows positive experiences in treatment. The patient leaves the group, finishes university and gains employment, while still maintaining friendly contact with the other group members.

## Conclusion

According to the experiences mentioned in the Clinical vignettes above, psychodynamic group psychotherapy is the method of choice in the therapeutic approach to the young population suffering from psychosis and to their family members. Over time, the RIPEPP programme (Restek-Petrović, et al., 2012; Restek-Petrović and Filipčić, 2016) has been added to, changed, and bettered, in accordance with the experiences gained, inhouse research, new knowledge from the literature, and from feedback from programme members (both patients and their family members).

# References

Addington, J. and Addington, D. (2001) Impact of an early psychosis program on substance use. *Psychiatric Rehabilitation Journal,* 25, 60–67.

Birchwood, M. and Fiorillo, A. (2000) The critical period of early intervention. *Psychiatric Rehabilitation Skills,* 4, 182–198.

Foulkes, S.H. (1977) *Therapeutic Group Analysis.* New York: International Universities Press.

Gonzáles de Chávez, M. (2009) 'Group psychotherapy and schizophrenia' in Y.O. Alanen, M. Gonzáles de Chávez, A-L.S. Silver and B. Martindale (Eds), *Psychotherapeutic Approaches to Schizophrenia Psychoses.* London: Routledge.

Kanas, N. (1996) Group therapy with schizophrenics: A review of controlled studies. *International Journal of Group Psychotherapy,* 36, 339–351.

Restek-Petrović, B. (2004) 'Grupna klima kao pokazatelj uspješnosti liječenja dugotrajne grupne psihoterapije psihoza' [Group climate as an indicator of effectiveness in long-term group psychotherapy of psychoses']. Doctoral thesis for the Faculty of Medicine, Zagreb.

Restek-Petrović, B. (2008) 'Grupna psihoterapija psihoza u ambulantnim uvjetima' ['Group psychotherary of psychosis for outpatients'] in E. Klain (Ed), *Grupna analiza: analitička grupna psihoterapija* [*Group Analysis: Analytical group psychotherapy*]. Zagreb: Medicinska naklada.

Restek-Petrović, B., Bogović, A., Mihanović M., Grah, M., et al. (2014) Changes in aspects of cognitive functioning in young patients with schizophrenia during group psychodynamic psychotherapy: A preliminary study. *Nordic Journal of Psychiatry,* 68, 333–340.

Restek-Petrović, B. and Filipčić, I. (2016) *Rana intervencija kod psihotičnih poremećaja* [*Early Interventions in Psychotic Disorders*]. Zagreb: Medicinska naklada.

Restek-Petrović, B., Gregurek, R., Petrović, R., Orešković-Krezler, N., et al. (2016) Characteristics of the group process in the long-term psychodynamic group psycho-therapy for patients with psychosis. *International Journal of Group Psychotherapy,* 66, 132–143.

Restek-Petrović, B., Mihanović, M., Grah, M., Molnar, S., et al. (2012) Early intervention program for psychotic disorders at the Psychiatric hospital 'Sveti Ivan'. *Psychiatria Danubina,* 24(3), 323–332.

Restek-Petrović, B., Orešković-Krezler, N., Mihanović M. and Štrkalj-Ivezić, S. (2008) 'Grupna psihoterapija u rehabilitaciji psihotičnih bolesnika' ['Group psychotherapy in the rehabilitation of psychotic patients'] in V. Jukić and Z. Pisk (Eds) *Psihoterapija: Škole i psihoterapijski pravci u Hrvatskoj danas* [*Psychotherapy: Schools and psychotherapy in Croatia today*]. Zagreb: Medicinska naklada.

Schermer, V.L. and Pines, M. (1999) *Group Psychotherapy of the Psychoses: Concepts, interventions and contexts.* London: Jessica Kingsley.

Urlić, I. (1999). 'The therapist's role in the group treatment of psychotic patients and outpatients' in V.L. Schermer and M. Pines (Eds), *Group Psychotherapy of Psychoses: Concepts, interventions and contexts.* London: Jessica Kingsley.

Winnicott, D.W. (1965) *The Maturational Process and the Facilitating Environment.* London: Hogarth Press.

Woodhead, G. (2008) 'Therapeutic group work for young people with first-episode psychosis' in J.F.M Gleeson, E. Killackey and H. Krstev (Eds), *Psychotherapies for the Psychoses: Theoretical, cultural and clinical integration.* New York: Routledge.

Yalom, I. and Leszcz, M. (2005) *The Theory and Practice of Group Psychotherapy.* New York: Basic Books.

# Chapter 15

# Group cognitive behavioural therapy for people experiencing psychosis

*Tania Lecomte*

## Introduction

Numerous trials have demonstrated that cognitive behaviour therapy for psychosis (CBTp) can reduce psychotic symptoms and the associated distress, as well as assisting individuals with psychosis in their recovery by improving their understanding and management of their mental health (Newton-Howes and Wood, 2013; Rathod, et al., 2008; Wykes, et al., 2008). Although most meta-analyses include some group CBTp trials, there have been more studies pertaining to individual CBTp than to group CBTp, and therefore less is known about the specific outcomes of group CBTp studies. In North America, for instance, group approaches for people with psychosis are much more common than in the UK, where CBTp was initially developed.

Group CBTp can either be general, focusing on distress and symptoms, or more specific (targeting a specific symptom such as voices, or an issue like self-esteem). Table 15.1 briefly describes the results of documented group CBTp studies and shows that overall, significant improvements were found in most studies, particularly regarding symptoms of psychosis but also in terms of self-esteem, coping and social functioning. Our own studies in group CBTp for early psychosis not only demonstrated improvements in symptoms, but also showed significant improvements in self-esteem and coping strategies, as well as social support above and beyond the level for participants who receive group skills training for symptom management (Lecomte, et al., 2008; Lecomte, Leclerc and Wykes, 2012). Only one group CBTp did not obtain positive results (see Table 15.1); a closer look at the study suggests that essential group therapeutic elements were not considered, which quite likely explains the poorer outcomes.

## Therapeutic elements of group CBTp

As with other group interventions, many of Yalom and Leszcz's (2005) essential therapeutic elements need to be present in group CBTp. For instance, normalisation (or universality) is one of the important steps in CBTp, i.e., to help clients feel less alienated by normalising their experience and getting them to realise that other people have had similar experiences (Kingdon and Turkington, 2005), and this is

*Table 15.1* Studies on group cognitive behaviour therapy for psychosis

|  | *Design* | *Aim* | *Outcomes* |
|---|---|---|---|
| Lecomte, et al. (1999) | RCT (exp vs. TAU), 24 group sessions (*n* = 95) | Improve self-esteem (Reasoner's developmental model) | Improved positive symptoms and coping strategies for exp group |
| Wykes, Parr and Landau (1999) | Pilot study, 6 group sessions (*n* = 21) | Coping with voices (cognitive strategies) | Diminished perception of voice power, diminished distress, improved coping |
| Leclerc, et al. (2000) | RCT (exp vs. TAU), 24 group sessions (*n* = 99) | Improve stress management (Lazarus' model) | Improved positive symptoms, self-esteem and hygiene for exp group |
| Chadwick, et al. (2009) | Pilot study, 8 group sessions (*n* = 22) | Diminish distress with voices | Diminished power of voice and feelings of control by voice |
| Granholm, et al. (2005) | RCT (exp vs. TAU), 24 group sessions (*n* = 76) | Combined CBT and social skills training to improve functioning in older patients | No effects on symptoms; improved functioning, coping and insight for exp group |
| Wykes, et al. (2005a, 2005b) | RCT (exp vs. TAU), 7 group sessions (*n* = 85) | Improve coping with voices and functioning | Effects on hallucinations only in the exp groups with more expert therapists; improvements in social functioning (exp only) |
| Barrowclough, et al. (2006) | RCT (exp vs. TAU), 18 group sessions (*n* = 113) | Improve positive symptoms | No effects on symptoms; only improvements on hopelessness and self-esteem |
| Landa, et al. (2006) | Pilot study, 13 group sessions (*n* = 6) | Improve paranoia (CBTp) | Diminished conviction in paranoid delusion, diminished distress |
| McLeod, et al. (2007) | Small RCT (exp vs. TAU), 8 group sessions (*n* = 20) | Diminish voices, improve coping with voices (CBT) | Diminished frequency and power of voices for exp group |

Notes
RCT: randomised control trial
exp vs. TAU: experienced groups vs. therapy as usual

easier to accomplish in a group context. Similarly, socialisation is central – the group format helps to overcome social isolation, which is one of the most prevalent consequences of psychosis. Social isolation, either being linked to social anxiety, paranoia, feelings of social incompetence, negative symptoms, or to stigma linked to having a mental illness, has severe consequences on the individual's integration in society. Group CBTp offers the opportunity to interact with others in a safe and nonjudgemental setting, and therefore to practice social skills and even to create friendships. In a CBTp context, the group participants help each other by suggesting alternatives to other members' beliefs, or by trying each other's coping strategies – which is also known as interpersonal learning.

For people with psychosis, group cohesion can take up to six sessions to build, and translates into feelings of belonging, sympathy and empathy for each other, as well as interpersonal learning and social support. A recent study by our team found that group cohesion strongly predicts improvements in symptoms and self-esteem in group CBTp – a strong cohesion offers the safety net required to dare to try new behaviours or to modify one's perceptions (Lecomte, et al., 2015; Lecomte, Leclerc and Wykes, 2018).

Group CBTp is time limited, and therefore aims at quickly offering a safe environment to participants, which is obtained via the use of a workbook that participants receive at the first session. As such, participants not only know what to expect, making them feel safe, but they can also peruse the themes of sessions to come and write their personal notes and thoughts at each session, which also helps to improve retention. In a previous study, the use of a workbook was in fact mentioned by many of the participants as one of the preferred aspects of the intervention, along with learning from the other group members (Spidel, Lecomte and Leclerc, 2006).

Group CBTp is extremely task focused in the sense that sessions have specific purposes that are translated into concrete discussion themes and active tasks during the sessions. Although recommended between sessions, homework is not the only practice time during group CBTp. In fact, each session is designed to encourage participants to work on their issues, to grasp new concepts, and to discover new coping strategies by different means (e.g., working individually, in pairs or everyone together). The sessions are designed to follow the single-session model, meaning that each session is complete and targets a specific concept or theme. When each session is clearly defined, participants leave the session with a sense of accomplishment and of purpose, with a concrete experience in mind. Group CBTp also uses a goal-oriented approach, with participants in the group being considered first and foremost as people with potential, strengths and qualities. This helps to foster the necessary self-confidence needed to believe that they can achieve things in their lives, and that their illness does not decide who they are or what they can do. This is also reflected in the fact that medical terms are not used, and that symptom names or diagnoses are not considered important. By avoiding psychiatric diagnoses and vocabulary, group CBTp offers the chance for participants to use their own terms to describe their experiences. We also use models, such as the stress–vulnerability–competence model (Anthony and Liberman, 1986), that focuses on protective factors and the person's ability to gain control over his/her own mental health. In fact, group CBTp is so positively oriented that one of its essential therapeutic elements is to have a pleasurable experience. Although difficult experiences and themes are addressed, this is done carefully in order to ensure that participants leave each session feeling okay, or better than when they arrived. Also, the socialisation period planned at the end of each session allows for friendly conversations to occur, which encourages a positive end to the group CBTp experience.

## Structure of group CBTp: A manual

Our team carefully developed and validated the 24 sessions that are offered in our group CBTp manual (see Lecomte, Leclerc and Wykes, 2016) in order to focus on strengths and self-esteem, as well as on symptoms and difficulties. By introducing themes in a gradual way, stress is prevented, and learning and sharing is favoured. The manual was developed 17 years ago and has since been validated in large studies. It is currently used with people with psychosis in more than 15 countries. Most activities in the manual involve introducing the theme to be discussed, followed by open-ended questions, which participants answer by writing in their workbook before sharing their answers with the group. (Each answer is personal and participants are informed that there are no 'good' or 'bad' answers). Each activity ends with a recap of what was discussed and what people wish to remember about the session. This is followed by a socialisation period where a light snack is offered and people are welcome to stay and chat. The 24 activities in the manual are equally divided into 4 parts:

1   stress, and how it affects me;
2   testing hypotheses and looking for alternatives;
3   drugs, alcohol and how I feel;
4   coping and competence.

The first phase of the treatment involves nonthreatening interactions in order to develop a therapeutic alliance, without which no treatment is possible. In the group, the first session aims to simply introduce each other and ask where the clients are from, what they like to do, and what they are good at (therapists also actively participate and share their answers). The second session introduces the concept of stress (a nonthreatening and universal phenomenon), and participants are asked to rate their emotional, physical and behavioural reactions to stress. The third session addresses events, people, places and situations that might induce stress, and clients need to determine to which stressors they are particularly sensitive. By the fourth session, the clients are asked to describe their first hospitalisation or their first encounter with a psychiatrist, and to explain what they believe happened. By the fifth session, the stress–vulnerability–competence model, focusing on protective factors, is introduced and personalised. This is considered as part of the CBT formulation whereby participants agree to consider a new model to explain their difficulties. By writing down their specific vulnerabilities, their stressors and their emotional and behavioural consequences of the interaction between the stressors and the vulnerability, participants make the model their own. The clients discover that they can actively work on building more and better protective factors, whereas they cannot easily control their vulnerability or the stress in their lives. Many of the protective factors are addressed in the CBTp workbook, and the participants are informed that they will be working on these during the following sessions.

The individual CBT formulation can also be found at other moments in the manual, particularly at session seven when the A–B–Cs of CBT are explained. By understanding how perceptions of events, not the events themselves, influence one's behaviours and emotions, participants learn how to see their own beliefs under a new light, and hence they become able to modify their reactions to stressful situations. Various exercises are used in order to reflect this link; for example, watching a movie excerpt, then generating multiple explanations for given situations, and eventually applying this to their own lives. For a more detailed description of the 24 sessions covered in the manual and how to conduct the group, see Lecomte, Leclerc and Wykes (2016).

Group CBTp does not solely focus on psychotic symptoms. In fact, participants can choose to work on any distressing thought, which can be interpersonal in nature (e.g., I feel lonely), or linked to depression, anxiety or anger. The manual focuses on how to deal with various emotions, while also helping the participants to recognise their values, strengths and qualities. Given the high prevalence of these issues, substance abuse and suicidal ideation are also targeted during the group. The last section of the manual concentrates more on coping strategies and meeting one's goals.

Eager and briefly trained clinicians might be tempted to 'jump right in' and try to modify dysfunctional beliefs linked to psychotic symptoms from the first session, without really taking the time to build the alliance and cohesion or to truly understand the issues. Yet the structure and content of the workbook describes optimum pace and helps the clinician to avoid certain mistakes. With a pace of one theme per session, with specific open-ended questions to engage the clients, therapists can see the effects of incremental learning (and avoid addressing difficult issues too quickly). Some issues, such as distressing beliefs, suicidal thoughts or substance use or abuse, can be difficult to address and might deter clients from continuing the therapy if they feel that the sessions are emotionally too difficult. The fact that many sessions focus on self-esteem is not only for their uplifting effect; improving self-esteem is essential for individuals with psychosis. One of our studies demonstrated a clear loop-like interaction between improvements in symptoms and self-esteem (Lecomte, Leclerc and Wykes, 2018). In group CBTp, self-esteem is addressed in various ways: by setting weekly personal goals, determining positive qualities and values, modifying attributions to become more optimistic in life, and by discovering one's competence in coping with various thoughts, voices or stressors.

Much has been written about CBT techniques: how to use them, their efficacy, etc. Unfortunately, this has led to many clinicians viewing them as effective ingredients that can be used at random, or at any given moment in therapy (Lecomte and Lecomte, 2002). This manual-based intervention therefore helps the less-knowledgeable clinician to use appropriate techniques at appropriate moments. For instance, normalisation is introduced early; seeking alternatives and checking the facts features later; and exploring coping strategies and developing a staying-well plan (i.e., relapse prevention) are discussed toward the end of the therapy.

## Therapeutic skills needed to conduct group CBTp

Less knowledgeable therapists might think that CBTp is more about techniques and psychoeducation than about interpersonal processes. However, as with all group therapies, the group CBTp therapists need to constantly observe and address three levels:

1   *The group level:* keeping in mind the theme being covered by the group today; making sure the group as a whole is doing well (no one is left out and there is a good atmosphere, etc.).
2   *The interpersonal level:* creating parallels between participants; encouraging interactions and interpersonal help; recognising and addressing conflicts.
3   *The intrapersonal level:* helping each person to work on their personal issues; making sure the group and themes are meeting each person's needs.

Even when following a manual, various interactions are at play in a group and the group therapists need to stay alert in order to deal with the issues that might arise. The group and its participants might feel frustrated leaving the group if only one of the three levels was addressed during the entire session. This may be because the therapists spent all the time discussing individual issues for each person without linking their experiences to others, or only focused on interactions or the day's theme without allowing time for personal disclosure. Competent group CBTp therapists will keep these three levels in mind and will try to make sure that they have all been addressed, even if only briefly, during each session.

As with most therapies, the group therapists need to express warmth, understanding and empathy. It might seem challenging to demonstrate flexibility while using a structured manual with predetermined themes. Yet flexibility can mean finding ways of making links between a pressing issue that someone brings to the group and the theme planned for the session. A therapist also needs to be skilful, in the sense of using the CBTp skills or techniques well. This implies mastering the skill, for example using Socratic questioning appropriately by carefully bringing the participant to realise that there are missing elements of proof supporting his/her distressful belief. Being skilful also implies being able to use different skills according to the situation or to the participant's current need. The concept of timing includes both time management, such as organising the session in order to provide sufficient time to complete the planned activities, and timing of an intervention, which is more about saying or doing the right thing at the right moment.

Therapist creativity is also essential and it not only implies a degree of flexibility, but also means thinking outside the box. Creative therapists will use the group members' input and might propose new ideas or activities when things do not go as planned. Creative therapists do not get 'stuck' in difficult situations, instead often finding original ways of making the group work optimally. Competent group CBTp therapists do not run the sessions alone – they skilfully engage participants into collaborating with each other, helping each other in various ways during the group sessions. As such, the participants do not spend the sessions talking to the therapists but interact among themselves, as well as with the therapists. The therapists model effective collaboration by working well together, in co-therapy, and by sharing explanations and activities, while also guiding participants in their interactions.

## Training and clinical applications for group CBTp

Our team has developed an active, brief and intensive training programme in group CBTp that has demonstrated positive results in terms of actual application of the skills learned. The training was developed with two goals in mind: being brief enough that most mental health workers could attend (i.e., 2 days), and offering a canvas that closely resembles what running a group looks like in real life. For the brief workshop to be effective, learning on multiple levels is targeted, and more than one teaching method is used, including role plays. Three levels of knowledge are targeted in order to promote real change: *Know* (i.e., the actual content or conceptual information pertaining to group CBTp), *Know-How* (learning how to apply specific group CBTp skills) and *Know-How-To-Be* (adopting the values and philosophy of the approach).

As mentioned at the beginning of this chapter, various group CBTp modalities exist: some with specific symptom focus (e.g., voices: Wykes, et al., 2005a); and others developed for older or cognitively impaired participants (Granholm, et al., 2005). Our own group CBTp was initially designed for individuals who were considered 'early psychosis' (i.e., youth and young adults who recently experienced a first psychotic episode), and is therefore less symptom oriented and more recovery oriented than other groups. However, our group CBTp format has since been altered: it has been offered to people with longer histories of mental illness, often once a week instead of biweekly. It has also been offered in a briefer version for people during short hospital stays or in forensic settings, and a family/carer version has also been developed for family members (Leclerc and Lecomte, 2012). Overall, group CBTp is highly appreciated by its participants and consistently demonstrates its usefulness in helping people in their recovery by gaining a sense of empowerment over their mental illness and helping them to move forward and to meet new goals.

## References

Anthony, W.A. and Liberman, R.P. (1986) The practice of psychiatric rehabilitation: Historical, conceptual, and research base. *Schizophrenia Bulletin,* 12, 542–559.

Barrowclough, C., Haddock, G., Lobban, F., Jones, S., et al. (2006) Group cognitive-behavioural therapy for schizophrenia. Randomised controlled trial. *The British Journal of Psychiatry,* 189, 527–532.

Chadwick, P., Hughes, S., Russell, D., Russell, I., et al. (2009) Mindfulness groups for distressing voices and paranoia: A replication and randomized feasibility trial. *Behaviour and Cognitive Psychotherapy,* 37, 403–412.

Granholm, E., McQuaid, J.R., McClure, F.S., Auslander, L.A., et al. (2005) A randomized, controlled trial of cognitive behavioral social skills training for middle-aged and older outpatients with chronic schizophrenia. *American Journal of Psychiatry,* 162, 520–529.

Kingdon, D.G. and Turkington, D. (2005) *Cognitive Therapy of Schizophrenia.* New York: Guilford Press.

Landa, Y., Silverstein, S.M., Schwartz, F. and Savitz, A. (2006) Group cognitive behavioral therapy for delusions: Helping patients improve reality testing. *Journal of Contemporary Psychotherapy,* 36, 9–18.

Leclerc, C. and Lecomte, T. (2012) TCC pour premiers épisodes de psychose: Pourquoi la thérapie de groupe obtient les meilleurs résultats? [CBT for first episode of psychosis: Why does group therapy offer better results?] *Journal de Thérapie Comportementale et Cognitive,* 22, 104–110.

Leclerc, C., Lesage, A.D., Ricard, N., Lecomte, T., et al. (2000) Assessment of a new stress management module for persons with schizophrenia. *American Journal of Orthopsychiatry,* 3, 380–388.

Lecomte, T., Cyr, M., Lesage, A.D., Wilde, J.B., et al. (1999) Efficacy of a self-esteem module in the empowerment of individuals with chronic schizophrenia. *Journal of Nervous and Mental Diseases,* 187, 406–413.

Lecomte, T., Leclerc, C., Corbiere, M., Wykes, T., et al. (2008) Group cognitive behavior therapy or social skills training for individuals with a recent onset of psychosis? Results of a randomized controlled trial. *Journal of Nervous and Mental Diseases,* 196(12), 866–875.

Lecomte, T., Leclerc, C. and Wykes, T. (2012) Group CBT for early psychosis – Are there still benefits one year later? *International Journal of Group Psychotherapy,* 62, 309–322.

Lecomte, T., Leclerc, C. and Wykes, T. (2016) *Group CBT for Psychosis – A guidebook for clinicians.* New York: Oxford University Press.

Lecomte, T., Leclerc, C. and Wykes, T. (2018) Symptom fluctuations, self-esteem, and cohesion during group cognitive behaviour therapy for early psychosis. *Psychology and Psychotherapy,* 91, 15–26.

Lecomte, T., Leclerc, C., Wykes, T., Nicole, L., et al. (2015) Understanding process in group cognitive behaviour therapy for psychosis. *Psychology and Psychotherapy,* 88(2), 163–177.

Lecomte, T. and Lecomte, C. (2002) Towards uncovering robust principles of change inherent to CBT for psychosis. *American Journal of Orthopsychiatry,* 72, 50–57.

McLeod, T., Morris, M., Birchwood, M. and Dovey, A. (2007) Cognitive behavioural therapy group work with voice hearers. Part 1. *British Journal of Nursing,* 16(4), 248–252.

Newton-Howes, G. and Wood, R. (2013) Cognitive behavioural therapy and the psychopathology of schizophrenia: Systematic review and meta-analysis. *Psychology and Psychotherapy,* 86(2), 127–138.

Rathod, S., Kingdon, D., Weiden, P. and Turkington, D. (2008) Cognitive-behavioral therapy for medication-resistant schizophrenia: A review. *Journal of Psychiatric Practice,* 14(1), 22–33.

Spidel, A., Lecomte, T. and Leclerc, C. (2006) Community implementation successes and challenges of a cognitive-behavior therapy group for individuals with a first episode of psychosis. *Journal of Contemporary Psychotherapy,* 36, 51–58.

Wykes, T., Hayward, P., Thomas, N., Green, N., et al. (2005a) What are the effects of group cognitive behaviour therapy for voices? A randomised control trial. *Schizophrenia Research,* 77(2–3), 201–210.

Wykes, T., Hayward, P., Thomas, N., Green, N., et al. (2005b) What are the effects of group cognitive behaviour therapy for voices? A randomised control trial. *Schizophrenia Research,* 77, 201–210.

Wykes, T., Parr, A.-M. and Landau, S. (1999) Group treatment of auditory hallucinations. *The British Journal of Psychiatry,* 175, 180–185.

Wykes, T., Steel, C., Everitt, B. and Tarrier, N. (2008) Cognitive behavior therapy for schizophrenia: Effect sizes, clinical models, and methodological rigor. *Schizophrenia Bulletin,* 34(3), 523–537.

Yalom, I.D. and Leszcz, M. (2005) *The Theory and Practice of Group Psychotherapy,* 5th edition. New York: Basic Books.

# Chapter 16

# Multi-family groups and psychosis

## A systemic approach

*Val Jackson*

This chapter aims to give readers an outline of the development of multi-family groups, an understanding of the rationale for multi-family groups, and to describe in more detail the groups run by the author, in the hope that readers will want to 'have a go'. It is hoped to convey the passion, enjoyment and trepidation that accompanied the author as she developed this way of working within the Early Intervention in Psychosis service in Leeds, West Yorkshire, UK (Jackson and Elks, 2007; Jackson and Gupta, 2010).

## The development of multi-family groups

The idea of working with families experiencing long-term mental health problems began in the 1940s primarily in the US, but it was Laqueur's work in the 1950s and 60s that led to the concept of multi-family therapy (MFT) (Asen, 2002). The initial aim was to improve the conditions on psychiatric wards where invasive clinical procedures, isolated patients and staff suffering from burn-out were common. Laqueur and his colleagues invited families onto the wards in order to bring new ideas to institutionalised ways of working. What was learned from this 'experiment' was that the exchange of ideas and experiences between families enabled them to learn from each other. Influenced by Bateson's theories of restricted feedback within a closed system (Bateson, 1972), Laqueur described the creation of multiple perspectives when several families came together, thereby challenging the dominant story (Cooklin, et al., 1976). His team noticed the impact of shared experiences, mutual support, constructive criticism and a modelling of individual independence and identity when in the presence of other families experiencing similar situations. The idea of a dominant story restricting the development of a self-identity is also reflected in more recent models of systemic practices, such as narrative therapy (White, 2007).

Much later, in the 1980s, McFarlane developed a substantial programme of psychoeducational MFT in the US for those diagnosed with schizophrenia. The description of schizophrenia as a chronic illness biological in nature was aimed at reducing the blame or guilt with which families would often present. Within this framework, there was little need for psychological 'insight'. Families were presented with information about the illness and services, and a problem-solving approach aimed to challenge dysfunctional ways of coping. The model also emphasised early and sustained contact with families, support to overcome challenges, the lowering of expectations, stress management, and social and employment needs. McFarlane's model was a long-term approach, lasting between 1–4 years. Outcomes demonstrated that the model led to lower relapse rates, increased employment and improved family relationships (McFarlane, 2002).

MFT was first used in English day hospitals in the 1970s when R.D. Laing's antipsychiatry ideas were prevalent and psychosis was predominantly thought to be the product of families. Initially, MFT was integrated into the general treatment plan until the Marlborough model developed as a distinct model (Asen, Dawson and McHugh, 2001; Cooklin and Asen, 2012) at the Maudsley Hospital in London. The advantages to the Marlborough model was that it was more effective and cheaper than treatment as usual (Asen and Scholz, 2010), and it was proven to be particularly effective with eating disorders. In the early days, the model combined systemic and psychoanalytical approaches, but the interpretative aspect of the latter proved to be more of an obstacle in this format. Influenced by Salvador Minuchin (1974), the groups developed a structure, using exercises that encouraged all participants to move between multiple roles, able to observe and learn from different positions. Therapists became conveners, orchestrating the activities. They also experimented with a reflecting team in a structured attempt to facilitate faster learning. The model was based on the principle that families and the relationships within them were a source of knowledge and skills, and the structured opportunities to share, reflect and observe others facilitated change. Building on these systemic principles of the Marlborough model, family therapists Asen and Scholz (2010) described the difficulties that individuals and families struggled with in reflecting on their own situations in the midst of personal conflict and distress, and at the same time were able to be sensitive and to advise other families confronted with similar difficulties. They aimed to utilise this finding in a safe environment characterised by mutual sharing, transparency and understanding. It seemed likely that positioning the family simultaneously as expert and as an observer of others, facilitated an important opportunity for stepping back and reflecting on their own situation leading to a new approach for the family, whilst increasing their own feeling of self-worth.

Although specific systematic data on the therapeutic outcomes of systemic MFT is limited, there are unpublished outcome studies that demonstrate the acceptability and usefulness of the approach (Asen and Scholz, 2010), particularly if running groups based around a common problem or theme (Asen, 2002). Evidence for MFTs using a systemic approach with psychosis is particularly scarce, especially in the UK. The available evidence is limited to long-term projects (1–4 years) and all the literature describes sustained interventions lasting several months or even years.

The multi-family groups carried out in the Leeds Early Intervention in Psychosis service for young people aged between 14 and 34 years during their first episode of psychosis also drew on systemic principles, but were planned as brief workshops over a period of 3 or 4 weeks. Families were encouraged to support and learn from each other, not only by observation of new perspectives from outside their own networks, but also by acknowledgment of each other's existing strengths and skills. This appeared to reduce defensiveness and to increase sharing and openness to new ideas.

## The structure of the Leeds workshops

Workshops were held twice a year using a variety of formats. All had an introductory evening, followed by further evenings or whole days 2 to 3 weeks later. Different formats were tried due to the difficulty of some family members being able to commit to consecutive days, but none of the workshops lasted more than 15 hours in total. However, it was observed that workshops run on consecutive days created a stronger connection between the families, which increased their ability to share. These connections continued for many months, if not years, after the workshops.

The minimum requirement for professional staff was two co-facilitators (family therapists) and two other support workers. Sometimes young children would attend without prior knowledge and it was always useful to have a worker who could play with them if adults needed time to reflect. The support workers also played a crucial role in observing individuals, particularly those who may be distressed and unable to find a voice to express this.

We chose different venues depending on availability and cost. Break-off rooms and a kitchen area where we could prepare food were useful. Sometimes participants were asked to bring a dish for a shared lunch, another time pizzas were ordered. A venue with a café on site and a children's farm attracted the largest number of participants, with 23 people attending from 8 families. Attendance varied considerably with representation from 3–10 families, ranging from 1–8 people per family. This could be a lone parent or whole families with aunts, uncles, grandparents, siblings and friends. The client was always encouraged to participate, but there was no requirement that whole families should attend. Each workshop used a similar format of structured exercises, which seemed to create a sense of safety for the group, and thus to aid individuals coming together for the first time to talk about a very difficult subject.

### Engaging families

Using flyers and phone calls, the Early Intervention service workers were encouraged to invite every client and their families in their case load. It became apparent that workers who had participated in a previous workshop became good salespersons for future workshops. Prior to the workshop, the co-facilitators visited families unknown to them at home two or three times. In addition, an introductory evening invited families to learn more about the workshop, the underlying service, philosophy about psychosis (an expression of something for which there had been no language: Seikkula and Arnkil, 2006), and a basic exercise to demonstrate what they might expect. The space between the introductory evening and the workshop also gave extra time to recruit more families.

### Aims of the workshop

Every workshop used structured exercises based on the following three stages and aims. A full description of these exercises and many more can be found in Asen and Scholz (2010).

#### 1: Strengthening family members' knowledge and confidence

These exercises helped individuals to get to know each other in a safe environment. They were also aimed at reducing the self-doubt, guilt and anxiety that many families experience, as well as trying to answer the many questions that needed answers for them.

*Example:* WHAT WE KNOW. Small groups, either random or gender specific (mothers, fathers etc.) created posters based on their knowledge of a chosen topic, e.g., cannabis, hearing voices, or how life changes. These were then presented to, and discussed by, the whole group (see Figure 16.1).

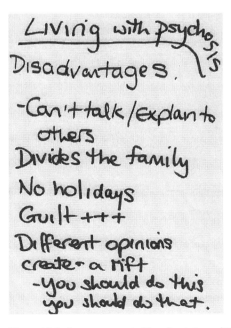

Figure 16.1 A poster created by clients in multi-family group therapy.

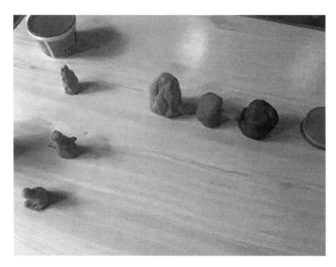

*Figure 16.2* A family group, as represented in Plasticine, created by clients in multi-family group therapy.

### 2: Exploring family relationships

These exercises enabled families to reflect on their situation through the eyes of other members of their own family and of the other group members. Being able to take a step back and view their situation as an 'observer' frequently resulted in surprising new perspectives.

*Example:* FAMILY SCULPTS. Family groups chose a medium to represent themselves (e.g., Lego blocks or Plasticine), and placed 'individuals' in relation to other family members, both in the present time and where they would prefer to be in future. Sometimes, young people would be invited to take a lead for this exercise, with parents observing. These were then discussed with the whole group (see Figure 16.2).

### 3: Reflecting on the future

As the last exercise of the day, it was hoped that families would take away a more positive view of their situation, focusing on what they have learned from their experiences and how this could influence the future.

*Example:* LETTER TO PSYCHOSIS. Individuals wrote an anonymous letter describing the positive effects of living with psychotic experiences. These were then chosen randomly by each person and read to the whole group (see Figure 16.3).

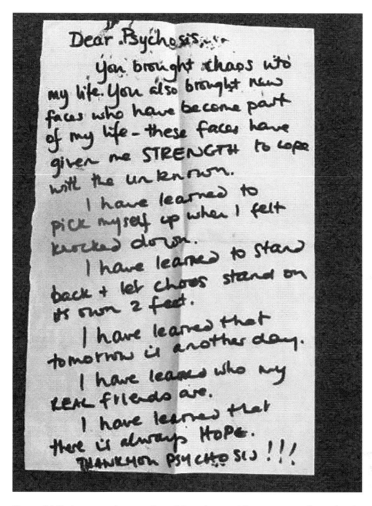

*Figure 16.3* An open letter, describing the positive aspects of psychosis, written by clients in multi-family group therapy.

### Clinical vignettes: Letters to psychosis

*Dear Psychosis*

You bought chaos into my life. You also brought new faces who have become part of my life – these faces have given me STRENGTH to cope with the unknown. I have learned to pick myself up when I felt knocked down. I have learned to stand back and let chaos stand on its own 2 feet.

I have learned that tomorrow is another day. I have learned who my real friends are. I have learned that there is always HOPE. THANK YOU PSYCHOSIS!!!

*Dear Psychosis*
You came as a bit of a shock. I'd heard about you but I didn't know you'd be so hard to deal with. I didn't think I'd end up with a flat in Leeds. I never thought I'd take up running along the canal or telling everybody I met all about you – so I learned their stories too. You've taught me that I can be a good Dad and a good husband. You've made me feel useful. You've helped me to stop walking around all day feeling sorry for myself. You've shown me how good my workmates are. And you've introduced me to lots of young, noisy, fun-loving kids. You've pulled my family closer together. So thanks. ×

*Dear Psychosis*
I learned how to express feelings more.

*Dear Psychosis*
I don't know why you made my son sick but it's made me stronger, also opened up my eyes to the little mistakes that I didn't realise were hurting him. Not telling him I love him. But now I tell him I love him all the time. So out of bad comes good, we are very close now.
  A grateful Mum

## Young people

Parents would often attend the workshops having been unable to persuade their son or daughter (the client) to attend. They were desperate to know what other young people thought about their psychosis, medication, cannabis, and so on. Sometimes it seemed as if the young people who did attend were being interrogated. As a consequence of this, the author met with several clients prior to the workshop without their families. Our service ran a regular group to bring younger clients together to participate in a variety of activities, so during one of these the group was asked to create posters about what parents do well and what they could do less/more of, their thoughts on cannabis, and on medication, etc. These posters were shown to the families who attended the workshops to facilitate discussions.

## Flexibility

Responding to the different needs during the day was crucial. This meant having at least two or three exercises planned at any one time. During one workshop it became apparent that none of the planned exercises for the afternoon would meet the expectations and needs of the group, so the lunch break provided an opportunity for the co-facilitators to make a new plan. Families were increasingly invited to take a more active role, so that a parent or a young person would take a lead on discussions, talking about their own experiences or suggesting exercises. Despite all the efforts to have confirmed numbers, there were always more or less people attending than expected and the workers would be asked to support an exercise if numbers were too high or too low.

## Evaluations

Each workshop was evaluated using an adapted SCORE (Stratton, et al., 2010). Individuals completed the same questionnaire at the start and at the end of each workshop. They were asked to rate each question from 1–5, in which 1 described their family very well and 5 did not describe them at all (see Figure 16.4).

Data from the questionnaires for two separate workshops was analysed independently with the following results (see Figure 16.5): a lower score indicates an improvement.

Individuals were also asked to rate how helpful the workshop had been in achieving their goal for their family (see Figure 16.6).

Although the numbers involved with the evaluation were very small, there is a clear indication that even a workshop as short as one day can enable families to move on with their lives. The challenge for the Early Intervention service staff was observing families who appeared to be struggling with life at home, but not having

| For each line, would you say *this describes our family*: | 1 Describes us: Very well | 2 Describes us: Well | 3 Describes us: Partly | 4 Describes us: Not well | 5 Describes us: Not at all |
|---|---|---|---|---|---|
| 1 In my family we talk to each other about things which matter to us | | | | | |
| 2 I understand everything that happens in our family | | | | | |
| 3 We trust each other | | | | | |
| 4 When one of us is upset they get looked after within the family | | | | | |
| 5 We are good at finding new ways to deal with things that are difficult | | | | | |
| 6 We have hope for the future of our family | | | | | |
| 7 My family feels a safe place to be | | | | | |

*Figure 16.4* The SCORE questionnaire, as used to evaluate multi-family group therapy.

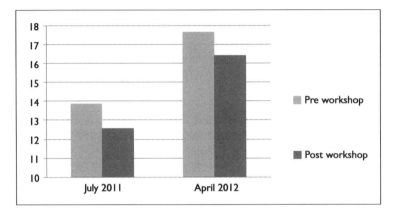

*Figure 16.5* Total average scores for questions 1 to 7 in the SCORE questionnaire, as used to evaluate multi-family group therapy.

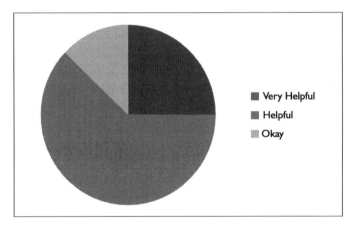

*Figure 16.6* Rating how helpful the workshop has been for each individual, as used to evaluate multi-family group therapy.

the resources available to offer further support. It became apparent that some families needed to be seen as a single unit, and a mixture of single-family sessions and MFT groups were often the most beneficial, as well as individual client sessions. Often these families had previously refused individual family therapy sessions, but attendance at these workshops encouraged them to seek further help.

## Summary

The purpose of this chapter was to give a background for the development of multi-family groups with psychosis, and to describe a basic short-term format with the hope that readers will be encouraged to run their own workshops. Although hard work, the workshops provided an ideal opportunity for workers to learn from the families, whose skills and resources were a constant source of inspiration. In addition there was always fun, laughter, and occasionally tears.

## References

Asen, E. (2002) Multiple family therapy: An overview. *Journal of Family Therapy,* 24, 3–16.

Asen, E., Dawson, N. and McHugh B. (2001) *Multiple Family Therapy: The Marlborough Model and its wider applications.* London: Karnac Books.

Asen, E. and Scholz, M. (2010) *Multi-Family Therapy: Concepts and techniques.* London: Routledge.

Bateson, G. (1972) *Steps to an Ecology of Mind.* Chicago: University of Chicago Press.

Cooklin, A. and Asen, E. (2012) Talking heads: Alan Cooklin and Eia Asen reflect on the history of the multifamily model at the Marlborough Family Service in London. *Context,* October, 3–7.

Cooklin, A., Asen, E., Mannings, C., Costa-Caballero, M., et al. (1976) 'Multiple family therapy' in P.J. Guerin (Ed), *Family Therapy: Theory and practice.* New York: Gardner.

Jackson, V. and Elks, G. (2007) Family intervention and psychosis: The story of the continuing development of family intervention in Aspire, Leeds, Early Intervention in Psychosis service (EIP). *Context,* 93, 17–18.

Jackson, V. and Gupta, A. (2010) The home-based model of family intervention in early psychosis. *Context,* 110, 39–43.

McFarlane, W.R. (2002) *Multifamily Groups in the Treatment of Severe Psychiatric Disorders.* New York: Guilford Press.

Minuchin, S. (1974) *Families and Family Therapy.* London: Tavistock.

Seikkula, J. and Arnkil, T. (2006) *Dialogical Meetings in Social Networks.* London: Karnac Books.

Stratton, P., Bland, J., Janes, E. and Lask, J. (2010) Developing an indicator of family function and a practicable outcome measure for systemic family and couple therapy: the SCORE. *Journal of Family Therapy,* 32(3), 232–258.

White, M. (2007) *Maps of Narrative Practice.* New York: Norton.

# Chapter 17

# A Moroccan multi-family group

## An example of cooperation with members of a minority group

*Margreet de Pater, Truus van den Brink*

## Introduction

People all over the world suffer from poverty, climate changes and war. Yet this is not the case everywhere. People in some countries are more lucky: most of them earn a decent wage and enjoy good healthcare and possibilities for education. A minority of people is very rich: the eight richest people possess as much money as 3.6 billion of the poorest people. So it is no wonder that people want to move from their own poor or/and unsafe country to a rich peaceful country. They pay a price, however: the loss of social connection. A similar price is also paid by people from the lower class in the recipient country, who have to live with the foreigners. They no longer recognise their old trusted neighbourhood, and they feel surrounded by people who speak a foreign language. Even small interaction problems cannot be solved by communication. This feeling of loss and insecurity becomes the basis for hate and mistrust, between all groups. In this climate, children, especially adolescents, who explore the world outside their family boundaries and often test the limits, are not able to thrive because the village that is needed to raise a child is unsafe.

## Social fragmentation, migration and psychosis

The fragmentation of neighbourhoods reflects itself in the statistics of psychosis. Allardyce and colleagues (2005) found a correlation between the number of hospital admissions for first-episode psychosis and defragmented neighbourhoods. The incidence of psychosis is also consistently higher in first and second generation migrants, and it is also higher than in the country of origin (Boydell, et al., 2001; Cantor-Graae and Selten, 2005). People who migrate from developed countries are less likely to suffer from psychosis. When a country chooses who is welcome and who is not (e.g., Australia), the incidence of psychosis is less than average (Selten, 2017). Also, living with people of the same migrant group in a neighbourhood has a protecting effect. Veling (2008) found that psychosis is more likely to occur for people who are living alone amidst other ethnic groups.

## Moroccans in the Netherlands

From the 1960s, Moroccan men left France to work in the Dutch mines (Blessing, 2004), where working conditions were better. In France, workers did not want dirty, poorly paid jobs; but in the Netherlands, Dutch workers were more assertive and demanded more pay and better conditions. Many Dutch companies went to Morocco to recruit workers. Among these Moroccan men, there was a high percentage of Berber people from the Rif mountains. This may have been because they were uneducated, many unable to read or write, or perhaps it was because King Hassan II encouraged the rebellious Berber people to leave. Berber (called 'barbarians' by the Romans) call themselves Amazigh, meaning 'free people'. Although they have a long history of brave battles against the Romans and other invaders, much of this history is now forgotten by most people of the Rif.

After a few years, the fathers who went to the Netherlands fetched their families because life was better. However, this situation had a disadvantage: fathers, who had been heroes in the family, now had low status jobs, and this often made it difficult to exercise authority, especially over their sons (Yildirim, van der Valk and Ajarai, 2016). Second generation male Moroccan youngsters have an especially bad name in the Netherlands: they are overrepresented in crime statistics, and they roam in the streets shouting insults at Dutch girls. This bad name hurts their brothers and sisters who are then unable to find a decent job. A circle of discrimination and crime has evolved, making life worse for Moroccans.

### Psychosis among Moroccan migrants

The incidence of psychosis (schizophrenia) among Moroccan inhabitants of the Netherlands is four to eight times higher than among originally Dutch or Turkish inhabitants, and among inhabitants of Morocco itself (Selten, et al., 2001). Moreover, the prognosis is unfavourable because Selten and colleagues believe that this higher incidence of schizophrenia could be connected to the low degree of structure in the Dutch–Moroccan community.

This prognosis appears to tally with the experiences of Moroccan family members, patients and social workers that we have come to know. Contact with the Dutch community is often painful. For young people, contact with their peers – Moroccan included – is also difficult. Conflicts between groups of Moroccans are sometimes worse than in Morocco itself. Sometimes they are completely unable to understand each other, because some speak Berber and others speak Arabic. In addition, there is a difference between Berbers from the north and Berbers from the south. According to the Moroccan parents and social workers that we have come to know, more Moroccans than Turkish migrants are integrated into the Dutch community. However, this makes the Moroccan community itself more disintegrated. The difference between the Moroccan and the Turkish population group is that the latter were more strongly organised at the time of immigration. Turkish people bought their goods in Turkish shops and had their own associations and networks. In this way, the Turks have been better able to protect their own people.[1]

## The development of a multi-family group for Moroccans

Having many Moroccan patients, we heard about these problems in the Moroccan community in the Netherlands. We then decided to do a pilot project in the form of a multi-family group (MFG), specifically for Moroccan people.

### Preparation

We invited two Moroccan fathers of our patients to have input as regards how the project should be organised. In the Netherlands, these two men occupy prominent positions in the field of social assistance to Moroccans. They were attracted by the idea that the MFG approach imitates a village community, although they did stipulate the need for separate men's and women's groups. In the villages where they came from, women from the same extended family group spent a lot of time together, and the same applied to men (Vries and Smits, 2005). Also, in some traditional families, women are not allowed to have contact with men who are strangers. We agreed to this condition, judging that otherwise a number of family members would not attend. Discussing problems between male and female family members would not be possible in this set-up, but usually this had taken place earlier in talks with the separate families. The chief aim was to form neighbourly relations.

Representatives from the family association Ypsilon were pleased with the start-up of a MFG, because so far they had not succeeded in reaching Moroccan family members. A Moroccan community worker from the Lombok district, Ahmed Essoussi, and a Moroccan psychologist, Laila Assa, were designated as group leaders. To liaise with various teams of the Zeist Regional Psychiatric Centre, a female social worker, Marijke Verhoeven, and a male case manager, Emile Rutger, were also involved. A psychiatrist was present in both groups. A prevention worker, Annemarie Feddes, organised consultations between the coaches to develop and coordinate the men's and women's groups and was responsible for organisational preconditions and reporting.

### Methodological adjustments

Besides forming separate men's and women's groups, we introduced other changes into the method. According to McFarlane (2002), a successful MFG lasts for 3 years. Our managers gave us a year to test whether the MFG was viable; after this time, its continuation was uncertain. Most of the participants could not read, so that information had to be communicated verbally. First, we would give a general account of how schizophrenia could impact on the family. Then we would present a list of themes to which the families themselves could add. We expected that, at a later stage, the group would feel safe enough for participants to introduce their own problems, questions and doubts. We also planned to invite speakers: an imam, Ypsilon and the Interaction Foundation (Kuipers, 2003).

### Recruitment

We thought that a preliminary meeting would be enough to recruit members, because most patients and families already knew us well. However, this assumption was wrong. Together with Ahmed Essoussi or Laila Assa, the Moroccan group leaders, I visited the candidates at their homes. Those prepared to receive us – which most were – also came to the group. Those who did not (always) come, pleaded transport and health problems. There were in fact transport problems: the bus connection was sometimes poor and the traditional clothing of some older women made it dangerous for them to cycle. For other women, it was difficult to take the right tram because they could not read the destination. I therefore gave a lift to three women from Nieuwegein, who found their way back by asking directions. Even when we had organised transport for two older women, they still failed to attend: their husbands said a little shyly that Moroccan men have less influence over their wives than Dutch people think.

### Composition of the groups

The common factor connecting the men's and women's groups was that all participants had long been struggling with psychosis in the family. There were also marked differences. The men's group contained older men with crocheted hats, but also elegantly dressed and highly educated younger men. Some found it very hard to talk about the problems at home; others were quite frank from the outset. There were men of Berber–Moroccan and of Arabic–Moroccan origin.

Initially, patients did not take part, because by their own account they had had their fill of psychiatry for the time being. Twice, at the invitation of a father, a patient from another family visited the group and made a constructive contribution. Among the women were single mothers who were bitter about the husbands who left them, but also a mother who indicated that solving family problems together had brought her closer to her partner. Some women barely left the house and could neither read nor write; others had good jobs. Some members had enthusiastically started to attend citizenship classes. Two female patients came along with their mothers and listened quietly. Another woman was both mother and patient and could clearly articulate the patient's perspective. One day two emancipated sisters suddenly turned up at the meeting and gave advice to their own and other mothers. On one occasion, the female interpreter brought her mother along.

### First experiences

In the beginning, it was perhaps the interpreters who played a decisive role in the eventual success. With our permission, they did not stick to their role and talked about other groups in which they had acted as interpreters and about their own emancipatory experiences. In addition, the two men who had taken part in the preparations were pioneers. One of them told how he had learned to coach his son with great patience instead of always disciplining him. The other had a more politically coloured role: he indicated that the Moroccan community lacks cohesion in the Netherlands due to the fact that people come from different regions in Morocco. With each subgroup speaking its own dialect and Moroccans (gradually) integrating into the Netherlands, the community shows a fragmented picture. Often the families did know each other, but were too ashamed to talk to each other about problems in their family. The time had come, he said, to break the silence. The wives of these men formed the heart of the women's group. One woman was an example for integrating into the Netherlands by speaking the language and moving freely; the other had a more traditional but also dignified personality. Both, in very different ways, had found solutions to the problem of dealing with their children's illness.

### Women's group

Beyond our expectations, the women quickly grew to trust each other. As they shared their experiences, they also raised emancipatory issues: for instance, urging each other to come by public transport so that their husbands did not have to bring them. They talked about their work and the courses they were following. From the list of themes, they immediately singled out the toughest subject: the issue of the patient marrying and starting a family. Opinions were divided. A more traditional mother had arranged her daughter's marriage with the latter's complete consent. Another mother would support her son, who was doing well, if he found a girl, but he had to build a life of his own. Some mothers were against the patient getting married and starting a family. Others expected that a partner would help their son to get better. The group leaders talked about their experiences: sometimes the marriage of a patient works out, but often it fails, because the role of partner and parent is very demanding for people with psychosis.

Another recurrent theme was: 'How involved should you be with your sick family member?' One mother asked the other women for advice: could she go to Morocco without her son? The women were unanimous in their opinion that she should stay. For her, this tipped the balance the other way and she decided to go on her own anyway! Some sons threatened their mothers with violence in order to get money to buy marijuana. The group discussed the dilemma. On the one hand, you want to protect your son: you do not want to see him homeless or hungry. On the other hand, you also need to protect yourself – and the constraint of clear rules can be of benefit. In general, the women learned to be firmer.

## Men's group

The men were mainly motivated to promote the interests of their sons/brothers, and so marriage was discussed in a different way. With the others' approval, one man asked whether we could issue a statement making it easier for them to bring over a marriage partner to the Netherlands and find housing.[2] We indicated our reluctance to help them in this way. Of course, we had heard that the older generations of Moroccans had some good experience with arranged marriages. Often partners knew each other from early youth, and although the relationship did not start with passion, couples gradually managed to forge a love bond. Yet did the same apply to this situation, with one partner seriously ill and the other in Morocco? Perhaps the Moroccan from Morocco would use the patient to enter the Netherlands, marry him, and then file for divorce? A father made it clear to us that the chance of abuse is actually smaller in the case of arranged marriages. Moreover, the Moroccan family code, 'El Moudawana', has been drastically revised under the new king. For instance, marriage partners are nowadays obliged to appear before a notary and submit a health certificate. We finally said that we would have to talk to the young couple ourselves before any undertaking.

The men wanted to stand up for their sons or brothers in other ways too. One patient was well known to the police, because they kept on bringing him back to the clinic when he failed to meet the conditions of discharge. Despite knowing that he was a patient, suffering from psychosis, the police always asked for his identity papers, which he never had because he always tore up his passport. The police would then cuff him and give him a fine, which his father would pay out of his pension. Although the men agreed that some of their sons or brothers misbehaved, it was their strong impression that this group was treated worse by the police than others. They sent a letter to the mayor, and a father proposed to form a father's group that could advise the police. Besides promoting the interests of their families, the men also exchanged experiences and often asked the Moroccan group leader for advice after the meeting. In general, the men learned to treat their sick son or brother with more patience.

## Guests to the group

Male and female representatives of Ypsilon visited both groups. The group members and Ypsilon members recognised each other's problems in the discussions. The Moroccan group members were invited as a group to form a separate subsection of Ypsilon. The imam from our mental health service was a guest of the men's group. He confirmed what the men already knew: sometimes native healers provide support, but there are also frauds. For the most part, the imam's talk focused on what the Koran says about tending to the sick. He explained that this is a duty and concluded by stating that the men were doing good work and that Allah would help them.

In a later phase, board members of the Interaction Foundation (a family-driven foundation) talked about their interaction training in both the men's and women's groups. In a role play, the psychiatrist played a patient who announced his plan to assassinate President Bush. This led to a lively discussion, especially in the women's group. Additionally, the regional healthcare centre visited the groups to give out information about patient fundholding.

## Mediation by group leaders

Language problems often hampered communication between family members and staff, for all their best efforts. For instance, a patient asked through his father whether he could go back to taking tablets instead of getting injections. After contact with the case manager, the psychiatrist prescribed the tablets, but in a form that dissolves rapidly in the mouth. The father did not realise that they contained the same active substance, and therefore kept on repeating his request.

The group leaders, the prevention worker and a member of Ypsilon helped to alert the mayor of Zeist to the problems surrounding the police's conduct towards patients. He answered that the police would now settle for a copy of an ID card. We were disappointed about this, having hoped that the Zeist council would take this opportunity to sit down and talk with the fathers and brothers. However, the group members themselves were pleased with his proposal and brought the ID cards to the meetings to get them copied and plastic coated in our facility.

## Evaluation

The members of the group who took part in the oral evaluation were full of praise. However, an independent and reliable assessment would have required semi-structured interviews in the homes of all the (non-)participants, including the members of the family who were patients. We therefore report a few salient points only.

Our initial idea was that the men would be mainly interested in promoting their family's interests, but for two men this was not true. On this point they gave a mark of 7 instead of 9 (out of 10); their criticism was that there should be more room for exchanging experiences. The women would have liked some more practical support. The Moroccan group leaders noticed that the participants took far more responsibility for guiding the patients' behaviour than before. The Moroccan group leaders also saw themselves as an essential part of the group's success, due to the fact that they were available outside of the group. Although there were ideas about undertaking structured problem solving – a crucial element in MFG – by using video instructions or integrating techniques of the interaction course, these ideas failed to materialise.

## Termination of the group

For various urgent reasons, all the group leaders, with one exception, were replaced by colleagues.[3] The groups continued for 6 months as support groups. Most of the nuclear group continued to participate, but soon after the women from Nieuwegein stopped attending (daunted by the distance of the journey now that they were no longer getting a lift from the psychiatrist). A few patients joined the men's group and articulated their experience of being psychotic, which led to more understanding among other parents. In retrospect, the patients found the session very difficult. A patient's partner attended the women's group, but felt too much distance from the mothers and sisters.

The only female patient told the mothers how nice it had been to think that she was the Virgin Mary. The mothers in the group understood, but had concerns for her children. Participation in the women's group decreased sharply, until the group leader, together with the interpreter, confronted the women: this kind of erratic behaviour was not typical of today's Moroccan culture. Could the women speak to their group members? After this they all returned. Unfortunately, the management decided that the costs of the MFG outweighed the benefits; a decision regretted by the participants.

### The progress of patients and family members

What became of the patients?[4] One man succeeded in keeping his job and remaining psychosis-free. The man who wanted to kill President Bush decided to take Zyprexa. Another accepted a depot and then adjusted his chaotic lifestyle. He now gets more support from his father and treats his mother more rationally. One man no longer upsets his parents with a litany of physical complaints and will soon move into independent accommodation. Another man will soon be discharged from the forensic institution where he stayed for years. However, the man who constantly tore up his passport keeps on protesting against his medication and his father, and regularly escapes from the ward. One man seemed briefly to be taking control over his life, but then returned to an inactive life in his mother's home. The arranged marriage of a woman never took place. Although her psychiatrist had signed a statement to help them find a house, the husband-to-be withdrew. After a crisis she recovered on a slightly higher level, but she only goes out to visit the shopping centre. One woman attempts a life without psychosis and tries harder to look after her children.

## Conclusion

Did the family group therapy contribute to recovery from psychosis? We cannot be sure, because the treatment was made up of many elements, and a MFG (according to McFarlane's methodology) never really coalesced. Yet, in the future, Moroccan family members will remain visible. Together with his daughter, a Moroccan man has set up a subdivision of Ypsilon, specifically for Moroccan family members. Most importantly, the emancipation of Moroccan people in the Netherlands makes progress, with Moroccan role models such as the Moroccan mayor of Rotterdam, Ahmed Aboutaleb, and the chair of parliament, Khadija Arib, both of whom are respected by all political groups.

## Notes

This chapter is modified from a version already published in *Netherlands Monthly Journal for Public Mental Health* (Pater-Zijlstra and Feddes, 2006), and in the book *De eenzaamheid van de psychose* (Pater-Zijlstra, 2012).

1   Selten recently said to me that he expected more Turkish young people to develop psychoses, because members of the next generation are more integrated, which will lead to the disintegration of the close-knit Turkish community in the Netherlands (personal communication, May 2005).
2   Nowadays in the Netherlands, income-level conditions restrict the introduction of marriage partners from abroad.
3   Margreet de Pater changed jobs; Laila Assa became pregnant, as did her successor; Ahmed Essousi became a town councilor; and Marijke Verhoeven had to limit her activities for health reasons.
4   The following information was received by telephone from persons in charge of the patients and family members who belonged to the nuclear group.

## References

Allardyce, J., Gilmour, H., Atkinson, J., Rapson, T., et al. (2005) Social fragmentation, deprivation and urbanicity: Relation to first-admission rates for psychoses. *The British Journal of Psychiatry,* 187, 401–406.
Blessing, M. (2004) 'De eerste Marokkanen in Nederland' ['The first Moroccans in the Netherlands']. Retrieved from: www.historischnieuwsblad.nl/nl/artikel/6581/de-eerste-marokkanen-in-nederland.html (accessed April 2018).
Boydell, J., van Os, J., McKenzie, K., Allardyce, J., et al. (2001) Incidence of schizophrenia in ethnic minorities in London: Ecological study into interactions with environment. *BMJ,* 323, 1336–1338.
Cantor-Graae, E. and Selten, J.P. (2005) Schizophrenia and migration: A meta-analysis and review. *American Journal of Psychiatry,* 162, 12–24.
Kuipers, T. (2003) Laat zien waar je staat, training van interactievaardigheden in de psychiatrie [Take your position: Training interaction skills in psychiatry]. *Maandblad Geestelijke volksgezondheid,* 58, 1137–1148.
McFarlane, W.R. (2002) *Multifamily Groups.* New York: Guilford Press.
Pater-Zijlstra, M.A. (2012) *De eenzaamheid van de psychose, de rol van veilige strijd bij het ontstaan en het herstel van een psychose* [*The Loneliness of Psychosis: The role of safe rebellion in the emergence and recovery of psychosis*]. Amsterdam: SWP.
Pater-Zijlstra, M.A. and Feddes, A. (2006) Marokkaanse familieleden uit de schaduw: een groep voor Marokkaanse patiënten met schizofrenie en hun naasten [Moroccan family members emerging from the shadow: A group of Moroccan patients with schizophrenia and their families]. *Journal of the Municipal Group of Valuers,* 61, 730–741.
Selten, J.P. (2017) 'Psychosen en migratie: een nieuwe meta-analyse' ['The relationship between psychosis and migration: A new meta-analysis']. Paper presented at the Voorjaarscongres, Maastricht.

Selten, J.P., Veen, N., Feller, W., Blom, J.D., et al. (2001) Incidence of psychotic disorders in immigrant groups to The Netherlands. *The British Journal of Psychiatry,* 178, 367–372.

Veling, W. (2008) 'Schizophrenia among ethnic minorities'. Rotterdam: Thesis Erasmus MC.

Vries, W.D. and Smits, K. (2005) Verdwaald in Nederland, het welbevinden van de eerste generatie Marokkaanse plattelandsmigranten [Lost in the Netherlands: The wellbeing of the first generation of Moroccan rural migrants]. *Journal of the Municipal Group of Valuers,* 1, 86–93.

Yildririm, S., van der Valk, I. and Ajarai, H. (2016). *Een halve eeuw in Nederland, de Marokkaanse arbeidsmigratie in 50 verhalen van Marokkaanse gastarbeiders en Nederlanders* [*Half a Century in the Netherlands: The Moroccan labour migration in 50 stories of Moroccan guest workers and Dutch people*]. Den Haag: Atlas Cultureel Centrum.

# Chapter 18

# The value of peer leadership in groups for persons with psychosis

## A programme for recovery and community health

*Larry Davidson, Anthony J. Pavlo,*
*Thomas Styron, Susan Mao, Ruth Firmin,*
*Richard Youins, Maria Edwards, Chyrell Bellamy*

The use of group psychotherapy for persons with psychotic disorders has diminished significantly in the US since the early 1980s, when studies began to show that intensive or investigative forms of psychodynamic treatment were not only ineffective for persons with psychosis, but in some cases could even be harmful (Gunderson, et al., 1984). For the most part, psychotherapy groups were replaced by psychoeducational and skills training groups; the most prevalent of which is the Illness Management and Recovery (IMR) approach developed by Kim Mueser and colleagues (2006), and disseminated by the US Substance Abuse and Mental Health Services Administration through its evidence-based practices initiative. In addition to IMR, there are a range of rehabilitative groups that focus on socialisation, recreation and finding safe ways to manage and recover from trauma, either due to earlier life experiences or to living in under-resourced and distressed urban communities (Najavits, 2002).

With the rapidly growing workforce of persons with lived experiences of mental illness and recovery being trained and hired to provide peer support, though, another new and exciting horizon has opened up for the development and evaluation of group interventions – those led by persons in recovery. The presence of such paid 'peers' (i.e., persons in recovery) within the mental health system is thought to bring with it several benefits for service users above and beyond the actual services they provide, including, most centrally, the instillation of hope and role modelling the possibility of recovery that their very existence makes tangible, as well as the experiential knowledge they can share based on their own struggles and successes in living with, and perhaps overcoming, a serious mental illness. Under this broad umbrella, there are two different types of groups in which peers play a leadership role: those led entirely by peers and those co-led by peer and non-peer mental health providers (e.g., clinicians). This chapter reviews the development of these two forms of group-based interventions for persons with psychosis in the US, beginning with those led solely by peers, and followed by those co-led by peers in a hybrid model that has been slower to evolve, but which appears promising nonetheless.

## Peer-led groups

The first groups led by persons in recovery in which persons with psychosis might participate were mutual support groups, which formed a central component of the Mental Health Consumer–Survivor Movement which began in earnest in the 1970s (Chamberlin, 1978, 1990). These groups were conceptualised as 'alternatives' to the conventional mental health system, and continue to thrive to this day as a meaningful source of support for people who find formal mental health services to be either antithetical to their recovery or inadequate to meet all of their needs. There is a substantial body of research on such groups, but much of this research took place decades ago and will not be reviewed here. Readers interested in this research are referred to our earlier work on this topic (for example, Davidson, et al., 1999).

The more recent developments in group interventions led by peers have emerged in the last two decades and have come about through the experiential knowledge such persons have acquired as they have entered into and pursued their own recovery. One prime example of such an approach that has garnered recognition internationally through The Copeland Center is the Wellness Recovery Action Planning (WRAP) approach developed by Mary Ellen Copeland in Vermont in the late 1990s in collaboration with others who were in recovery (Copeland, 2008). WRAP is a strength-based approach to practicing self-care on a day-to-day basis that includes advanced planning for potential crises, which can be developed and utilised on an individual basis, but which is often taught in groups. There has been some empirical evidence suggesting that WRAP improves self-care and advocacy, and achieves a number of recovery-oriented outcome domains (Cook, et al., 2010, 2012; Fukui, et al., 2011; Starnino, et al., 2010).

A second approach for which there is not yet as much empirical evidence, but which is just beginning to generate broader interest, is the *Pathways to Recovery* workbook developed by Priscilla Ridgway and colleagues at the University of Kansas (Ridgway, et al., 2002). This self-described 'strengths recovery self-help workbook' uses the metaphor of a journey to introduce and explore the notion of recovery in relation to serious mental illness, with chapters on such topics as 'gearing up', 'setting the course', 'moving forward', and 'rest stops and travel tips', among others. While it, too, could be used on an individual basis, it is often offered as a self-help tool in a group format, and has been the subject of two studies thus far; one in which the group was peer-led (Fukui, et al., 2010) and one in which the group was co-led by peers and counsellors (Green, et al., 2013), both finding positive outcomes in recovery-oriented domains.

For the purpose of this chapter, we would also like to highlight a third approach in which peer facilitators of groups may be trained, even though this approach has not spawned its own groups *per se*. This is the approach of Intentional Peer Support (IPS) developed by Shery Mead (2005), and it offers a framework within which peer-led groups utilising different self-help tools might be developed. That is, while WRAP and *Pathways to Recovery* may be offered in a group format – and may even focus on what members can do to increase their social support outside of the group – they primarily focus on what persons with serious mental illnesses can do on their own behalf to self-manage their condition, and their overall life, as they pursue recovery. IPS, on the other hand, is a model of peer support that addresses how relationships between individuals are essential to everyday life and healing in nature, reinforcing the mechanisms of mutuality *between* group members to promote beneficial effects for members. In this respect, we find IPS to be more consistent with a purely peer-based perspective, as it stresses reciprocity in relationships in ways in which it would be inappropriate, if not impossible, for clinicians to participate, at least in their role as clinicians (they could participate as private individuals, but not in their organisational capacity as clinical practitioners). These are groups in which we could say that it is the 'peerness' itself of the leaders and members that provides the most salutary effects, rather than any specific self-help curriculum that the peer happens to be offering.

IPS differs from traditional clinical or service relationships by not beginning with the core assumption that there is 'a problem' that has brought the person to the group. Instead, peer leaders are taught to listen for how and why each person has learned to make sense of their own experiences, and then to use their relationships to explore new ways of seeing, thinking and doing that the member may not have tried in the past. IPS is also sensitive to the prevalence of trauma in the lives of persons with mental illnesses, avoiding the implication that the person has done something 'wrong' that requires treatment. Instead, IPS asks the person about *what has happened* to them and explores alternative ways of dealing with what has happened. Rather than a focus on what the person needs to stop or avoid doing, or what symptoms the person needs to be rid of, peer leaders encourage group members to move towards what and where they would like to be in their lives. Within this context, connecting to others (and reconnecting to others following disruptions) lie at the heart of the healing process, and offers a potent antidote both to trauma and to mental illness among group members. In our experience, when peer group leaders approach their work from this relational perspective, building on the mutuality that exists among all group members (including themselves), tools like WRAP and *Pathways to Recovery* become even more effective in promoting and sustaining recovery.

## Hybrid groups

We have already mentioned one hybrid group that was co-led by a peer and a counsellor and utilised the *Pathways to Recovery* curriculum (Green, et al., 2013). Our team has been experimenting with hybrid groups since the mid-1990s, and has developed a 'home group' model that we think maximises the contributions both of the peer and of the clinician co-leader by differentiating and conceptualising their roles as complementary.

The role of the peer is to instill hope by providing visible evidence of, and role modelling the reality of, recovery. The peer also shares his or her accumulated experiential, or 'insider', knowledge of how to both survive and to overcome mental illness, substance use, and an everyday life that has been salvaged from the ravages of trauma and traumatising social conditions such as poverty, prolonged unemployment, exposure to violence, and discrimination. Nothing has proven to be as potent a response to stigma and discrimination as being introduced to a living, breathing example of a person who has shattered the negative stereotypes associated with having a mental illness or an addiction. By their very presence in the group, peer leaders already challenge members to imagine and come to believe in the possibility of having better or fuller lives than those restricted to the confines of mental health and substance use programmes. Finally, peer leaders who are trained in IPS and/or in person-centred care planning (Tondora, et al., 2014), can offer to accompany or support group members in their care planning meetings with other members of their care team.

On the other hand, the clinician's role in the home group model builds on the clinician's professional training and accrued expertise in both group facilitation, and illness and stress self-management. The first focus of the clinician's work is to facilitate connections between the group members and to help to establish a culture of mutual support, using process-oriented interventions to highlight commonalities and shared experiences, and modelling and eliciting members to provide encouragement and feedback to each other. Within this context of peer support, the clinician can then also elicit topics or issues of interest among the members and, when appropriate, provide materials and resources to stimulate further discussion and perhaps offer self-care tools. In this respect, components of WRAP and *Pathways to Recovery* can be used to educate members about adaptive coping strategies and self-care techniques. The clinician can also provide material resources and concrete assistance that are available to deal with benefits/entitlements issues, housing, employment, or social and leisure activities in the community that members might like to explore. In contrast to a traditional process-oriented psychotherapy group, members are encouraged to explore such activities together outside of the group – with or without the support of the peer leader – and are generally encouraged to rely on each other for support outside of the group. A prominent and explicit goal of the home group is therefore to facilitate an expansion of each member's social network, with members trading telephone numbers and email addresses, and offering both practical and emotional support to each other in their daily lives.

The name 'home group' was chosen to reflect that one of the main aims of the group was to provide the members a 'home base' from which to establish a foundation both inside the mental health system (for accessing other healthcare and social services), and in their local community (to establish a sense of belonging). Members are encouraged to take risks to explore additional services (e.g., medication and primary care), additional supports (e.g., supported education and employment), and naturally occurring social and recreational activities in the community (e.g., joining a faith community, romantic dating or attending sporting events, etc.). Members can then return to the group to process their efforts. They also are provided with support to navigate the various systems and community venues, both by the peer co-leader and by fellow group members. Finally, the members are encouraged to 'own' the group as theirs and to take an active role in shaping how they spend their time together. To facilitate this sense of ownership and elicit member feedback on a regular basis, the last section of each group is spent asking each individual to grade how useful the group has been on this particular day on a scale of 1– 10, with 10 being the best score. When members grade a group as not so helpful (i.e., 1–7), the co-leaders ask the members how it could be made more helpful in the future. This end-of-group 'check-in' mirrors how the group opens each week, with each member rating 1–10 for how bad/difficult (1) to good/enjoyable (10) their previous week has been. The group lasts 1 hour and 15 minutes: the check-in typically takes about 20 minutes; the middle 40 or so minutes is spent discussing issues the group chooses, based either on issues generated during the initial check-in or carried over from previous weeks; and the feedback takes about 15 minutes.

Much of the practical support provided derives from the members' own experiences with managing their own behavioural health conditions and navigating the medical and social service systems, and is modelled initially by the peer co-leader. In this way, practical advice and social–emotional support are often intertwined.

## Clinical vignette 18.1

A group member was concerned about a medication side effect. The peer co-leader encouraged him to discuss the issue with his doctor, and helped him in the preparation of questions, by looking up information on the internet. The other group members then normalised his concerns by discussing their own adverse reactions to medication changes. One group member also shared information about a new service at the mental health centre, saying: 'I am going to this group on medication education next Tuesday and I want you to come with me'.

One of the more striking instances of both practical support and generosity came when one woman disclosed to the group that she was having difficulty setting boundaries with family members who were behaving in problematic ways and that she feared she would become homeless. Group members asked her a few questions to understand her difficulties better; several members drew from their own, similar, experiences and expressed empathy and encouragement; and one member offered to share her own, limited resources: 'If I get my new place like I'm supposed to,' she said, 'I'll have an extra room. You can stay with me: I'm not going to let you be on the street.'

## Clinical vignette 18.2

At a group meeting being held on a Thursday afternoon, one member expressed distress over a recent disappointment in her life and told the group that she was concerned about the upcoming weekend due to increasing suicidal ideation. In the past, when she felt this way and was about to embark on an unstructured and empty weekend (i.e., when she had no plans to see any one or do anything interesting), she would invariably end up in the hospital after presenting herself to the emergency room scared that she would hurt herself. This particular day she had no desire to spend her upcoming weekend in the hospital, but was having difficulty coming up with any other ways of how she might manage her distress and suicidal thoughts.

At this point, the peer co-leader asked the members if they had any suggestions. Another woman in the group shared that she, too, had no particular plans for the up-coming weekend and perhaps the two of them might have a 'sleep over' at her apartment, the way girls often do during their preteen and adolescent years. She had fond memories of those earlier times in her life, and was also feeling lonely and isolated. She then pointed out that it was autumn, and that traditional activities to do on weekends are to go apple picking and to make apple pies. She wondered if perhaps they could go on such an outing together. Other group members encouraged the pair to follow through on these plans, and to report back to the group the following week about how the weekend had gone.

After the group ended, the clinician co-leader met with the two women together, and assessed the first woman's degree of suicide risk. If she began to feel unsafe in the next few days, the plan was to contact the clinician through the agency's on-call system. However, the weekend passed without incident, and at the next meeting, the two women enthusiastically shared their stories of apple picking and pie baking with the group. As a result, the first woman discovered at least one alternative way of managing her distress and suicidal thoughts that did not result in a visit to the emergency room or admission to the hospital, while the second woman spent an enjoyable weekend with a new friend, feeling less alone in the world.

In these groups, the traditional understanding of therapeutic boundaries is transformed, based on the emphasis on reciprocity and the inclusion of a peer co-leader. Such basic human interactions (including physical contact) and gestures (such as helping to address members' basic needs), are incorporated into the group rather than prohibited from it.

## Clinical vignette 18.3

During one group, a member arrived late and was looking through the window of the door to the group room. The peer co-leader excitedly waved at her to come inside and the group welcomed her once she entered the room. During her check-in she said: 'I really needed that'. When the clinician co-leader asked her what she meant, the member explained that she needed to be 'seen' and 'welcomed in'. She then tearfully explained that her doctor had recently told her that she needed to have a biopsy to determine whether or not she had cancer. While feeling 'too emotional' to attend her Alcoholics Anonymous meeting, she nonetheless came to her home group, 'to be with family . . . welcomed . . . hugged'. Following her comment, each group member and co-leader stood up, walked over, and gave her a hug.

## Clinical vignette 18.4

During a group check-in, a member rated her feelings as 3 (not very well). She explained to the group that she had not received a cheque from her guardian for the past 2 weeks and was unable to buy food or cigarettes. At this point the peer co-leader offered to loan her $5 from the tips he had made the previous night at a music gig. After some encouragement, the group member accepted the money and, with tears in her eyes, said: 'I love you. Thank you, Brother'. During check-out at the conclusion of the group, the member rated the effectiveness of the group at 10 (very helpful) and expressed gratitude to the group for their support.

While neat positive resolutions to members' problems or needs cannot always be reached, it is true to say that difficult situations, feelings and concerns can be lightened through sharing them with caring others.

## Clinical vignette 18.5

A group member talked about her relationships with her daughter and granddaughter. She told the group that she had been a 'negligent mother' while struggling with drug addiction and mental illness when her daughter was young and that this had damaged their relationship over time. She went on to describe having made every conceivable attempt to mend her relationship with her daughter, but that nothing seems to have worked.

She now experiences her daughter as disrespectful, often using profanity, and not abiding by her rules while living in her home. The group member expressed her despair to the group, which was met with silence. Slowly, group members began to share their complicated experiences with their own children. One woman spoke about her feeling of guilt related to her 'enabling' her son's substance use. Another group member shared about his relationship with his son, who had also witnessed his addiction as a child. This group member disclosed that he had not seen his son in 2 years. Another group member expressed to the group that she had accepted that she would not be able to mend her relationship with her daughter, and now instead focuses her energy on developing a strong bond of love with her granddaughter and helping to create a better life for her.

On this morning, there did not seem to be any solutions to specific problems, but group members connected through the similarities of their experiences. Their experiences had different shades and dimensions, but group members left saying that they felt less alone. At one member's suggestion, the group ended with the serenity prayer: 'God grant me the serenity to accept the things I cannot change, the courage to change the things I can, and the wisdom to know the difference'.

Table 18.1 summarises the various interventions utilised in the home group hybrid model in terms of their primary aims, during key areas of concern: from a position of social isolation to having adequate social support; from feeling demoralised to developing a sense of self-efficacy; and from being disengaged from care to engaging productively in treatment. These primary areas of concern were identified through previous research as posing major barriers to recovery among persons with serious mental illnesses who experienced multiple admissions to psychiatric hospitals and/or multiple emergency room visits (Davidson, et al., 1997). Within this context, preliminary evidence supporting the effectiveness of the home group approach for this population has shown increases in outpatient utilisation and social functioning, reductions in substance use, and more active involvement in self-care (Bellamy, Schmutte and Davidson, 2017).

## Conclusion

Far from having complete or definitive answers or models, we are just at the beginning stage of exploring the various ways in which peers – persons in recovery – can contribute in a meaningful and effective fashion to leading group interventions for persons with psychosis. We have witnessed first-hand the restorative impact that the presence of peers can have on persons with serious mental illnesses who have struggled for prolonged periods of time with the stigma, discrimination, demoralisation, and despair that come from receiving messages of hopelessness,

*Table 18.1* Interventions used in the home group model during key areas of concern

| From social isolation to social support | From demoralisation to self-efficacy | From disconnection to engagement in treatment |
| --- | --- | --- |
| 1 Assist group members to engage in social connections with other members:<br>— help members to share their experiences of social disconnection and isolation,<br>— encourage members to accompany each other on community explorations.<br>2 Facilitate and encourage specific acts of mutual support and reciprocity among group members:<br>— encourage expressions of caring, camaraderie and friendship among members,<br>— assist members to recognise and respect social cues and personal boundaries in their interactions.<br>3 Facilitate local community outings and activities with group members:<br>— provide planning, financial support and transportation for once-weekly, local community outings led by peer-support staff,<br>— enhance members' independence, and familiarity and connections with affordable, local community activities and resources. | 1 Assist group members to recognise and share the problems they face and the changes that occur:<br>— encourage members' expressions of hope in the possibility of change and recovery,<br>— help members to share their struggles with constricted resources and help them to apply for needed assistance.<br>2 Facilitate participatory decision making and planning among group members:<br>— help members to recognise how their actions impact on the group and other members,<br>— encourage members to make specific plans for unstructured time, such as weekends.<br>3 Provide individually tailored, flexible support to group members experiencing crises:<br>— increase members' engagement and contact intensity,<br>— advocate for interdisciplinary team meetings to plan special support and outreach efforts. | 1 Encourage members to face symptoms and difficulties in relating, when these become evident in interactions of the group.<br>2 Help group members to recognise changes and improvements in their symptoms and problems.<br>3 Connect group members with abstinence-based self-help groups for substance use:<br>— support members' engagement in these groups by rewarding with positive recognition,<br>— encourage members to connect with sponsors,<br>— facilitate group celebrations of milestones in recovery.<br>4 Facilitate the experience of group members as active partners in their care:<br>— help members to recognise their fears of medication side effects and stigma,<br>— train members in using the person-centred care planning tools,<br>— assist members to honestly face struggles between acquiescence and compliance,<br>— advocate for collaborative care planning between members and outpatient clinicians and other service agencies. |

| From social isolation to social support | From demoralisation to self-efficacy | From disconnection to engagement in treatment |
|---|---|---|
| 4 Create and maintain group celebrations:<br>— assist members to celebrate milestones in recovery and to maintain community tenure,<br>— enhance members' connections with seasonal rhythms, and with local events and celebrations. | 4 Facilitate the emergence and recognition of group members' natural interests:<br>— encourage members to state preferences and interests in participatory planning of community outings and group celebrations,<br>— help members to initiate activities with others who share their interests,<br>— recognise members' particular strengths, skills and natural leadership roles,<br>— recognise and encourage members to share their interests, motivate their initiative, and enhance engagement in activities. | 5 Provide outpatient clinicians with information about group members' daily lives and environment; their cultural, racial, ethnic, gender, religious identity; and their functional disabilities and strengths.<br>6 Consult with outpatient clinicians regarding frustration and demoralisation concerning group members' continuing difficulties. |

chronicity, and disappointment from a mental health system that engendered dependency and focused on maintenance as the best that life had to offer. These individuals have much to gain from exposure to tangible evidence and role models of recovery, and from the accumulated life experiences and associated wisdom that such persons have gained in both practical and social–emotional ways through their own struggles. What remains to be seen is if and how the value of these contributions might be adapted for, and offered to, persons earlier in the course of illness, such that they can avoid the considerable iatrogenic damage done to generations past. For this, new models and approaches may still need to be developed that can keep young people engaged in their lives and pursuing their dreams so that future re-integration efforts become unnecessary.

## References

Bellamy, C., Schmutte, T. and Davidson, L. (2017) An update on the growing evidence base for peer support. *Mental Health and Social Inclusion,* 21(3), 161–167.

Chamberlin, J. (1978) *On Our Own: Patient controlled alternatives to the mental health system.* New York: Haworth Press.

Chamberlin, J. (1990) The ex-patients movement: Where we've been and where we're going. *The Journal of Mind and Behaviour,* 11(3&4), 323–336.

Cook, J.A., Copeland, M.E., Corey, L., Buffington, E., et al. (2010) Developing the evidence base for peer-led services: Changes among participants following Wellness Recovery Action Planning (WRAP) education in two statewide initiatives. *Psychiatric Rehabilitation Journal,* 34(2), 113.

Cook, J.A., Copeland, M.E., Jonikas, J.A., Hamilton, M.M., et al. (2012) Results of a randomized controlled trial of mental illness self-management using Wellness Recovery Action Planning. *Schizophrenia Bulletin,* 38(4), 881–891.

Copeland, M.E. (2008) *The WRAP Story: First person accounts of personal and system recovery and transformation.* West Dummerston, VT: Peach Press.

Davidson, L., Chinman, M., Kloos, B., Weingarten, R., et al. (1999) Peer support among individuals with severe mental illness: A review of the evidence. *Clinical Psychology: Science and Practice,* 6, 165–187.

Davidson, L., Stayner, D., Lambert S., Smith, P., et al. (1997) Phenomenological and participatory research on schizophrenia: Recovering the person in theory and practice. *Journal of Social Issues,* 53, 767–784.

Fukui, S., Davidson, L.J., Holter, M.C. and Rapp, C.A. (2010) Pathways to Recovery (PTR): Impact of peer-led group participation on mental health recovery outcomes. *Psychiatric Rehabilitation Journal,* 34(1), 42–48.

Fukui, S., Starnino, V.R., Susana, M., Davidson, L.J., et al. (2011) Effect of Wellness Recovery Action Plan (WRAP) participation on psychiatric symptoms, sense of hope, and recovery. *Psychiatric Rehabilitation Journal,* 34(3), 214.

Green, C.A., Janoff, S.L., Yarborough, B.J.H. and Paulson, R.I. (2013) The recovery group project: Development of an intervention led jointly by peer and professional counselors. *Psychiatric Services,* 64, 1211–1217.

Gunderson, J.G., Frank, A.F., Katz, H.M., Vannicelli, M.L., et al. (1984) Effects of psychotherapy in schizophrenia: II. Comparative outcome of two forms of treatment. *Schizophrenia Bulletin,* 10, 564–598.

Mead, S. (2005) *Intentional Peer Support: An alternative approach.* Plainfield, NH: Fishery Mead Consulting.

Mueser, K.T., Meyer, P.S., Penn, D.L., Clancy, R., et al. (2006) The Illness Management and Recovery program: Rationale, development, and preliminary findings. *Schizophrenia Bulletin,* 52(1), S32–43.

Najavits, L. (2002) *Seeking Safety: A treatment manual for PTSD and substance abuse.* New York: Guilford Publications.

Ridgway, P.A., McDiarmid, D., Davidson, L., Bayes, J., et al. (2002) *Pathways to Recovery: A strengths recovery self-help workbook.* Lawrence, KS: University of Kansas School of Social Work.

Starnino, V.R., Mariscal, S., Holter, M.C., Davidson, L.J., et al. (2010) Outcomes of an illness self-management group using Wellness Recovery Action Planning. *Psychiatric Rehabilitation Journal,* 34(1), 57.

Tondora, J., Miller, R., Slade, M. and Davidson, L. (2014) *Partnering for Recovery in Mental Health: A practical guide to person-centered planning.* London: Wiley-Blackwell.

Chapter 19

# Voice-hearing groups

Empowering ourselves –
The Hearing Voices Movement

*Olga Runciman*

The Hearing Voices Movement (HVM), which has existed for more than 25 years in the UK, 12 years in Denmark, and can be found in more than 30 other countries, was inspired by the innovative research of Marius Romme and Sandra Escher (1993, 2000). Their research advocated a radical new approach and a profound shift in perspective on the symptoms traditionally associated with schizophrenia – hearing voices.

> Treating patients' experiences as meaningful is profoundly threatening to the medical model of madness which is dependent on meaninglessness or the supposition that lived lives are of secondary importance.
>
> (Runciman, 2013, p. 66)

The HVM has since evolved into a two-pronged movement.

## HVM: A protest movement

Firstly, HMV is a protest movement against the dominant psychiatric paradigm that states that hearing voices and having other unusual experiences is a primary symptom of schizophrenia. It further states that schizophrenia is a serious and debilitating brain disease for which there is no cure, but it can be managed by drugs. For example, if one is to look on a website such as the American Psychiatric Association, or another schizophrenia information website such as SIND (the Danish website for mental wellness), or a pharmaceutical website such as Lundbeck, the following will be a typical description of the symptoms of schizophrenia:

- voices, visions, smells and tactile experiences, viewed as hallucinations;
- delusions, or false beliefs as they are also colloquially known;
- negative symptoms referring to emotional blunting;
- cognitive issues often referred to as disorganised thinking.

Likewise, the causes of schizophrenia are typically listed as: (1) it is genetic and inheritable; (2) the result of environmental influences in the form of viruses, malnutrition and/or autoimmune disturbances; and (3) ascribed to disturbances in the neurotransmitter system of the brain. This is why neuroleptics are seen as beneficial. However, for a voice hearer, this is seen as both meaningless and dehumanising.

Another major symptom of schizophrenia is often referred to as anosognosia, or a lack of 'illness insight', when a person diagnosed as schizophrenic rejects the label and the fact that they are ill, making them seem to be resistant to treatment. Anosognosia is believed to be found in 57% to 98% of all schizophrenic patients (Lehrer and Lorenz, 2014). The HVM challenges this by introducing the meaningfulness of life stories and the consequences of trauma as evidence that the label of 'illness' is untenable. Romme and colleagues (2009) established that the voices were meaningful and made sense when viewed in conjunction with the traumatic life events that provoked them. Furthermore, research has shown that at least 75% of voices hearers have had some traumatic experience connected to their voices (Read, et al., 2005; Johnstone, 2007; Hammersley, et al., 2008; Moskowitz and Corstens, 2008).

## HVM: A self-help group methodology

The second aim for HVM will be the focus for the rest of this chapter. HVM, by being an influential grassroots movement which openly critiques traditional psychiatry's relational roles of 'passive, recipient patient' and 'dominant, expert clinician', has created a strong self-help tradition where people can meet in a safe place in their groups and share experiences,

> without the threat of censorship, loss of liberty, or forced medication, a common feature of disclosure in traditional psychiatric settings.
>
> (Dillon, 2011)

HVM have therefore researched, developed and published their own methodologies, techniques and narratives, as separate from psychiatry, to help those who have problems with their voices, visions, etc. Voices are seen in these groups as a survival strategy, pointing at past and present problems, often using the language of metaphors which represent emotions split-off from the self, and often telling tales of dreadful events – attacking and yet protecting the person's identity.

Trauma is a dominant theme, from sexual abuse, emotional neglect, physical abuse and bullying, and it becomes clear within these groups that these events play a profound role in the development of alternative beliefs/experiences. The purpose of the groups is not about getting rid of the voices, but about understanding their message(s) and changing the relationship so that the voices may become helpful and cease to be damaging. Thus, with the Hearing Voices groups, 'madness' is placed in a context where it can become accessible and understandable, which challenges those who view these experiences as irrational, or as symptoms of an underlying biological phenomenon.

## Description of a voice-hearing group

*As a voice hearer myself, I have been running groups for more than 10 years. Although one can view these groups through the lenses of diverse therapies, such as from a narrative perspective or open dialogue, it is the fact that it is the more-experienced voice hearers guiding the less-experienced to learn how to become a voice hearer; that is the game changer.*

The group described here is open and ongoing. There are presently four men and three women, with myself as the group facilitator. One of the men and one of the women come only sporadically, but the rest come regularly. Hearing voices is common for all of them, some members have visions, and one man experiences tactile sensations. For some, paranoia is also an issue.

To describe the role of the group facilitator (see also Bullimore, Crawford and Reeve, n.d.), it is easier to say what it is not. The facilitator is not responsible for the success or failure of the group, for keeping people happy, getting people interested, getting people there, or for making refreshments. In other words, the responsibility of the group rests with the group. However, the group has a clearly defined recovery-orientated perspective, promoting empowerment and the importance of creating one's own meaning and understanding, as well as acknowledging the member's own expertise within an accepting environment.

All members have been labelled schizophrenic, and are therefore one of the most marginalised and stigmatised groups of people that exist within the mental health system. What becomes clear when working with people labelled schizophrenic has been how devastating the actual label has been for that person's life. If looking at it from a narrative perspective, it is that which is deemed a problem that is the problem, rather than the person being the problem. However, for the person labelled schizophrenic, schizophrenia becomes all-encompassing and a problem in itself. This is true for the members of the group, for not only are they faced with the challenge of dealing with their voices, but they also have to face the everyday consequences of being marginalised and stigmatised. The label 'schizophrenia' is so powerful that many identify totally with their label and become 'schizophrenic'. It is this journey from *being* a schizophrenic to *becoming* a voice hearer that is the purpose of the group.

The journey in a Hearing Voices group, from being labelled schizophrenic to becoming a voice hearer, typically occurs in four stages, as described by anthropologist Sidsel Busch (2015), as well as occurring in my own experience in the groups and in my private practice. In the first step, group members are encouraged to give in to their voices, which in essence means to start actually listening to their voices. Often people have refused to listen or acknowledge what is being said by their voices. Frequently they are afraid or enraged by their voices, seeing them as disconnected from themselves, and therefore denying the things the voices say as having any relation to them. Members experience the voices as outside of themselves, saying that they are the CIA, demons, neighbours or family members, etc. Since this is the first time that members have truly listened to what is being said, they may initially feel overwhelmed. The second stage is when members start to try to identify the voices, to find out who they are, and to find meaning and interpret what the voices are actually saying. At the third stage, members begin to engage with the voices, to set limits, and to relate the voices to past and present triggers. Although we encourage people to give names to their voices and experiences early on, when they first come to the group, it is usually at this stage when members speak easily of them by name and gender, connecting them to themselves. By the fourth stage, the member is a voice hearer, who has become experienced with the voices, knows intuitively how to handle them, and is no longer afraid or controlled by them. The voices are now viewed as guides and sources of inspiration. For some, having understood their message and dealt with the issues that the voices represented, the voices disappear – but for many, however, this is not the case.

All of the group members have been, or are still, caught in problem-saturated stories that they have told themselves. Yet of even more consequence are the stories that society has told them about themselves, while also ostracising them from society. These stories are highly disabling and disempowering. Disenfranchised by society, many group members feel that there is no hope for the future and that they are spectators, watching the world go by.

Although the Hearing Voices group is a self-help group, and therefore not controlled by any form of therapeutic model, it is possible to relate elements in the group dynamic to therapeutic theories, such as the narrative form of psychotherapy. For example, the emphasis on the importance of life stories, and the language used when telling the stories (also an element in open dialogue), is crucial when trying to create meaning and understanding, along with hope for the future (Arnkil and Seikkula, 2006). Both open dialogue and narrative theory stress, above all, the importance of language in shaping people's realities. The group members need language to shape their realities because, being part of the psychiatric system, they are entrenched in a language *about* them, rather than *with* them, and where power, authority and expertise belong to the psychiatric system and not to themselves. From an open dialogue perspective, the way in which members perceive and experience themselves and their situations has been constructed through culturally mediated social interactions. This occurs because cultures are continually sending crucial messages through the use of language and stories about important concepts such as gender, race, class and, of course, health. In this way, personal and cultural beliefs about health are strongly influenced by the norms and standards of that particular society. Hence, within our society, hearing voices is socially undesirable and the symptom of a biological disease rather than something meaningful and intimately related to that person and their life story.

Another important aspect of the Hearing Voices groups is the recovery concept: the fact that people can, and do, recover. However, we are not referring to a traditional viewpoint of recovery, which is based on illness and cure. Instead, we refer to concepts such as empowerment, self-esteem, self-determination and respect. The recovery philosophy is based on the uniqueness of the individual, and therefore recovery for some will mean recovering from an illness, whereas for others, recovery is recovering from psychiatry. Others refuse to use the word 'recovery', feeling it has been colonised, and choosing instead to describe their experiences in different ways. This is reflected in the group, for there are those who believe in the illness model and are therefore compliant with the psychiatric belief system, and there are those who reject this model and experience the consequences of noncompliance.

One of the major themes of narrative therapy is that the person is not the problem; the problem is the problem. Therefore, a major focus in narrative therapy is on trying to separate the problem from the person. This is done through a process called externalisation, whereby the problem is placed outside of the person and back into a cultural context. Clients in narrative therapy are often encouraged to give their problem a name, so that they can refer to it in the third person and thereby separate and create distance between themselves and their problem. The focus is then to look at how the problem influences the client's life and the narrative that surrounds that problem (White, 2007).

From a narrative perspective, members in a Hearing Voices group could be described as not only having externalised their problems, but also as having externalised them so successfully that they have separated completely from them, and the focus in the group is to bring the problems (voices) home to where they belong as part of the person and their life. For example, some members give their voices names, and they are also able to describe how their problems, as represented by the voices, are affecting their everyday lives. Therefore, one could conclude that voice hearers are experts at externalisation, although this has not been explored in depth within the narrative therapy research. Yet multiple truths exist: other group members will not see their voices as part of them and their life stories, but instead consider them to be spiritual. These different meanings and understandings within a group are all valid, and they emphasise that the unique role of experienced voice hearers guiding the less experienced cannot be translated into treatment models, or copied and incorporated into the psychiatric system.

## Vignette 19.2

Philip is in his early 40s and began to hear voices for the first time when he was a child and then sporadically in his teenage years. It was in his late 20s that his voices began to invalidate his life and he sought help in the psychiatric system. However, it was only when he found the Hearing

Voices network and discovered that there was another way to approach his voices that made sense to him, that he was able to turn his life around.

Philip's childhood was filled with fear: he was exposed to neglect and violence, especially by his father. He also had vague memories, which were shadowy and diffuse, of something happening to him sexually by his father, which made him confused as to whether he could be gay. (In his case, being gay was not a problem, in contrast to another group member, who had an intense fear of being gay because he had been abused by men in his childhood, and thus associated loving men with paedophilia.) Philip was the youngest in a household of older sisters. He never felt that he had received much support from his sisters, especially after his parents died. They were very sceptical and critical of his decision to choose another route rather than the traditional psychiatric one.

When he first came to the Hearing Voices group, Philip had no idea who his voices were, having accepted psychiatry's explanation that they were not real, but a symptom of schizophrenia, and the solution was medication. In his case, medication had often been a help, but his quality of life had been impaired so that he often chose to have periods without medication, which then meant being bombarded by his voices. The Hearing Voices group revolutionised his life.

In the group, Philip discovered who his voices were and what they represented. They were his family members symbolising chapters in his childhood and his repressed emotions, especially of anger, that had been forbidden to him as a little boy. His most problematic voice was the voice of a little boy whom he discovered was actually himself. He had problems controlling the little boy who would easily become enraged when Philip's boundaries were crossed or when he was criticised. Philip was able to put down boundaries for his other voices, apportioning them with 2 hours of undivided attention every day, which meant they did not bother him the rest of the day. However, his little boy voice would not accept this and continued to turn up during the day. A breakthrough happened when a group member suggested that instead of fighting the little boy, Philip should change tactics and invite the little boy to be with him during the day. Philip did this and the relationship changed. The little boy stopped being so angry with Philip for constantly trying to keep him away. In conjunction with this changed relationship, Philip discovered that many times when the little boy reacted, he was reacting relevantly. In fact, he was reacting the way Philip wanted to react but which he had learned was forbidden and dangerous as a child. Philip discovered that, for him, his voices represented his repressed emotions and his inability to put down boundaries.

Today, Philip functions as a facilitator himself.

## Conclusion

In our experience as voice hearers, and as Busch (2015) states, the voice-hearing groups work because they strip away the dominant power structures found within psychiatry, and offer a space of true safety and normalisation. The major contributory factor in this success is that the experienced voice hearer guides the less-experienced. Inspired by the success of these groups, many well-meaning professionals wish to recreate these groups within psychiatry, but these fail because they are enmeshed in the dominant power structure of their workplace that sees voice hearers as schizophrenics. However, inspiration from the Hearing Voices Movement is leading to positive change, both for patients and for staff. Today, many professionals work alongside voice hearers in academia, research and every-day practice, resulting in a changing attitude that is questioning the traditional concept of schizophrenia.

## References

American Psychiatric Association: www.psychiatry.org/patients-families/schizophrenia/ what-is-schizophrenia (accessed May 2018).

Arnkil, T.E. and Seikkula, J. (2006) *Dialogical Meetings in Social Networks*. New York: Karnac Books.

Bullimore, P., Crawford, K. and Reeve, T. (n.d.) 'Starting and sustaining paranoia and hearing voices self-help groups – A facilitator's guide'. Pamphlet. Sheffield, UK: Asylum Books Limbrick Centre.

Busch, S. (2015) 'At blive og være stemmehører stemmehører: Et antropologisk studie af stemmehøring og læring i stemmehører bevægelsen i Danmark ' ['To become a voice hearer: An anthropological study of voice hearing and learning']. Ph.D. dissertation for the University of Copenhagen.

Dillon, J. (2011) 'The personal is political' in J. Moncrieff, M. Rapley and J. Dillon (Eds), *De-Medicalizing Misery: Psychiatry, psychology and the human condition*. London: Palgrave Macmillan.

Hammersley, P., Read, J., Woodall, S. and Dillon, J. (2008) Childhood trauma and psychosis: The genie is out of the bottle. *Journal of Psychological Trauma*, 6(2/3), 7–20.

Johnstone, L. (2007) Can trauma cause 'psychosis'? Revisiting (another) taboo subject. *Journal of Critical Psychology, Counseling and Psychotherapy*, 7(4), 211–220.

Lehrer, D.S. and Lorenz, J. (2014) Anosognosia in schizophrenia: Hidden in plain sight. *Innovations In Clinical Neuroscience*, 11(5 6), 10–17.

Lundbeck: www.lundbeck.com/global/brain-disorders/disease-areas/schizophrenia (accessed May 2018).

Moskowitz, A. and Corstens, D. (2008) Auditory hallucinations: Psychotic symptom or dissociative experience? *Journal of Psychological Trauma*, 6(2/3), 35–63.

Read, J., van Os, J., Morrisson, A.P. and Ross, C.A. (2005) Childhood trauma, psychosis and schizophrenia: A literature review with theoretical and practical implications. *Acta Psychiatrica Scandinavica*, 112(5), 330–350.

Romme, M. and Escher, S. (1993) *Accepting Voices*. London: MIND.

Romme, M. and Escher, S. (2000) *Making Sense of Voices: A guide for mental health professionals working with voice-hearers*. London: MIND.

Romme, M., Escher, S., Dillon, J., Corstens, D., et al. (2009) *Living with Voices: 50 Stories of Recovery.* UK: PCCS Books in association with Birmingham City University.

Runciman, O. (2013) 'Postpsychiatry's challenge to the chemical treatment of mental distress'. Thesis for the Department of Psychology, University of Copenhagen.

SIND: www.sind.dk/skizofreni1 (accessed May 2018).

White, M. (2007) *Maps of Narrative Practice.* London: Norton Professional Books.

# Chapter 20

# The group in arts therapies

## An additional therapeutic medium for working with psychosis

*Sheila Grandison*

In mental health care in the UK, the four arts therapies – art psychotherapy, dance movement psychotherapy, dramatherapy and music therapy – have developed a distinct place among other psychological therapies as evidence-based and highly valued interventions with service users.[1] As these therapies are not principally language based, they offer alternative channels of communication for interpersonal relating where talking therapies can struggle or even fail. Combining psychotherapeutic techniques with activity aimed at promoting creative expression, the arts therapies can provide a bridge to verbal dialogue. In focusing treatment directly on relational and interpersonal understanding, the use of groups and group work within the arts therapies is widespread. When delivered as group interventions in the NHS, the arts therapies are also efficient against the backdrop of increasing budgetary restraints in the public sector.

There is growing evidence for the use of groups in the arts therapies in both acute and community mental health settings. The updated 2014 guideline from the National Institute for Health and Care Excellence (NICE) for psychosis and schizophrenia in adults continues to recommend offering arts therapies 'to assist in promoting recovery, particularly in people with negative symptoms' (NICE, 2014, p. 31). Negative symptoms may be defined as emotional apathy, lack of motivation, poverty of speech, withdrawal and self-neglect, but their overwhelming effect is social isolation. The guideline also specifies that the arts therapies should be provided in groups, 'unless difficulties with acceptability and access and engagement indicate otherwise' (NICE, 2014, p. 25–26). Along with the broad aim of enabling people with psychosis to express themselves, is the more specific therapeutic challenge of 'helping people with psychosis to accept and understand feelings that may have emerged during the creative process [and] to experience themselves differently' (NICE, 2014, p. 25–26). With attacks on experiences of feeling, linking and relatedness central to psychotic functioning, how can the arts therapies provide empathic responses to those presenting with complex communication difficulties? Also: how can transformative change be tolerated, held and contained in a way that enables people with psychosis 'to experience themselves differently' and to develop new ways of relating to others?

Rooted in the premise that the group is where the currents of relationship between individual and group meet, arts therapies, along with the other psychological and sociotherapeutic group approaches and interventions, share the humane aim of decreasing individual isolation. Annie Rogers (2016) describes how psychosis, in particular, thrusts the individual into radical isolation, describing how words alone can be insufficient containers for powerful emotions and how:

> Many people lost in psychosis (for a short time or over a very long time) experience things that cannot be symbolized, spoken, or received by others.
>
> (Rogers, 2016, p.3)

It is in this area of the seemingly impenetrable where the arts therapies are perhaps best known, receiving non- and pre-verbal communication, engaging with it, and aiming to find through images, sound or movement, a dialogue with that which is not yet able to be expressed in words. For people struggling to find meaningful relatedness in the world of real people and the world of human relationships, art, drama, dance movement and music therapists endeavour to establish emotional contact by being in relation with them creatively.

Engagement can be a major obstacle in delivering psychological interventions. The arts therapies have been promoted as a means of helping people to engage in psychological treatment for those who have profound difficulty verbalising their feelings, thoughts and life experiences. As the arts therapies are commonly delivered in groups in the UK, they lend themselves to being used in multicultural settings in which many service users speak little English. Arts therapists working in London NHS Trusts confirm that consistently high numbers of service users attending arts therapies groups are from black and ethnic minority groups, with a high proportion of males with a diagnosis of psychosis engaging in them. The arts therapies therefore make a significant contribution to reducing fear, stigma and health inequalities in mental health care by increasing accessibility and extending group interventions to service users for whom English is not a first language, and who may be identified as 'difficult to reach', 'hard to engage' and unsuitable for the talking therapies. In turn, this has a positive impact on the wait times and capacity of wider psychological therapies services.

Each of the arts therapies has nonverbal interaction at the core of its approach for facilitating the expression of emotions through creative activity. Verbal communication may be opened and expanded through creative activities. Groups take place in specifically designed therapeutic environments suitable for creative activity, where each individual is helped to find their own unique starting point in the creative process and encouraged to explore the art materials, musical instruments or other props in the group with the support of the therapist. The therapist continues from where the service user begins, through relating musically, visually or through movement, in an interactive way. The creative forms made can then provide a bridge for talking in more depth in the group, where appropriate.

In acute settings, where there is a fast turnover of service users, arts therapists need to show quickly and effectively the benefit to service users of coming into an art or music therapy room. A first step may be just being in the room and accepting the art materials or musical instruments the therapist has to offer – having a look, trying out an instrument or a crayon – making use of 'other'. This acceptance is understood by arts therapists as a form of interpersonal engagement, conveying a level of willingness shown by the service user to communicate with another. The opening of a psychological window, no matter how small, may have been reached, enabling possible further interaction with the arts materials and engagement of the service user with the arts therapist. When working with acute states of mind in inpatient settings, these early pre-therapy stages are necessary for developing attachment. As Dratcu (2002, p. 81) points out, 'admission is likely to occur when there has been a failure in the patients' support network, formal or informal', which is a time when being with others in groups is experienced as being profoundly difficult and so help is needed in restoring interpersonal relating.

The practice of arts therapies mediates between concrete and symbolic ways of thinking. In art psychotherapy for example, the visual image made from the process of using the concrete art materials retains all the characteristics of human effort. For example, a crayon connecting with a piece of paper produces a range of distinct audio sounds that accompany the emergence of a visual image as the paper takes the mark-making. The sound of the crayon moving to and fro across the page as the hand moves from one area of the paper to another, the crayon's sound if pushed away urgently by the hand during the process, and the sound of the dif-ferentiation in rhythms and pressures given to the crayons as they make contact with the paper throughout the drawing process, all make for a combined audio-visual communication, as well as a somatic performance. The end embodied visual image, far from being static, preserves the invested energy and communicative endeavour. It comes alive again in the process of its reception by the art-therapist viewer. The visual image is a live intersubjective form. In her exposition of the life of pictures, Marion Lauschke (2014) can be understood as summarising what arts therapists refer to as the triangular therapeutic relationship – between art-maker, therapist, and the artwork made (be it visual, musical or physical). Of visual images, 'picture documents', Lauschke says:

> Although all symbolic forms originate in the transformation of states of psychosomatic arousal, picture documents have the greatest ability to preserve the invested energy [. . .] to discharge it during reception, acting as a stimulat-ing source of creativity. They can invite calm contemplation and pleasure in that which is unthreateningly alive, but they can also impose the re-experience or embodiment of their generative affect onto the beholder and cause an inten-sification of emotions. Pictures stand in a tension between these two poles.
>
> (Lauschke, 2014, p. 229–230)

Containing the uncontainable is how 'the aesthetic form is used in the arts therapies to contain and give meaning to patients' experience' (NICE, 2014, p. 25–26). Helping to organise experience can differ in each of the arts therapies. In music therapy, by introducing a change of rhythm or sound in a group improvisation, the music therapist can calm and modulate affect, whilst sustaining the creative potential for music-making. In art psychotherapy, the art therapist, when working with clients with avoidant relationship patterns, can help them to stay connected by shifting attention from interpersonal issues to the activity of art making (see Greenwood, 2012). In dramatherapy, action-oriented processes such as role play, mime and storytelling, can hold the narrative. Finally, in dance movement psychotherapy, interacting through movement enables service users to become aware of their interpersonal behaviour, allowing them to modify how they form and maintain relationships with others.

It is in the interplay of both psychic and creative dynamic processes at work in the arts therapies where the symbolic and the concrete are held simultaneously, and the work of strengthening, or creating, psychic structure lies. 'Art de-frags my brain, like a computer rearranging the files into different places', is how one service user described his experience of art making. However, working with psychosis in acute settings can bring about the risk of psychic assaults, as described by Gordon and Kirtchuk (2008, p. 7–8):

> The link (attachment) between the patient and other people; between the patient and his own thoughts, feelings, experiences and history; between the patient as an individual and the social group – including the ward milieu – to which he belongs: these links are all seriously disturbed, distorted, attacked or obliterated.

Working psychodynamically with psychosis, Maurizio Peciccia and Gaetano Benedetti (1998) recognised that many cases of psychoses are connected to a split between the symbiotic self, which links the person to others, and the separate self that differentiates the self from others. They developed a technique of communication with their patients using visual images, called progressive mirror drawing. Both therapist and patient made drawings on transparent sheets of paper, which could be superimposed on top of each other, joined together, and separated from each other, and could be used therefore as the concrete means for symbolic self–object differentiation. The drawings held the movement of symbiotic contact between the patient's and the therapist's drawings (overlapping, superimposing and joining) and the distancing from that contact (separating), with the therapeutic aim of integrating symbiotic and separate selves to counter the psychotic split. Through their mediation between concrete and symbolic ways of thinking, anxiety could be sufficiently alleviated to develop and sustain therapeutic engagement, and a particular form of containment is rendered in the arts therapies, one which is unthreateningly alive.

In arts therapies groups, the unconscious emotional life of the group is held in the core *visuality, musicality,* and *physicality* of the group's image, music and movement-driven narrative. How do we understand the relationship of the personal images, sounds and movements made by individuals in the group, to the group-as-a-whole communication? In arts therapies groups, therapeutic attention is given as much to the personal connections of, for example, hands on a drum or mark-making, as it is to group connections. Models and methods may vary across the arts therapies for facilitating group cohesion, with different levels of structure and direction from the therapist. Just as group analysis focuses on the individual and the whole group at the same time, particular attention is given to the adaptation in arts therapies groups of the Foulkesian group-analytic concepts of resonance and group matrix.

Of the first concept, Foulkes (1964, p. 292) defined the group matrix as:

> the hypothetical web of communication and relationship in a given group. It is the common shared ground which ultimately determines the meaning and significance of all events and upon which all communications and interpretations, verbal and non-verbal rest.

The concept of a living matrix was seen by Roberts (1996) as holding all 'the subtleties and delicacies [and] the complexity and vulnerability of living processes' within its web. Both individual and group mutually influence each other, with both the conscious and unconscious assumptions brought into the group carried within the connective tissue of the matrix. Group processes opposing the development of a living matrix were identified by Nitsun (1996) with his concept of the antigroup. The coexistence of the creative and destructive potential of groups is particularly pertinent to group arts therapies where, as in verbal group-analytic groups, both creative and destructive processes are at play, but where the concrete and symbolic manifestations of creativity and destructiveness can be either acted in, or acted out.

The second group-analytic concept of resonance is developed when the group as a whole 'seems to become highly charged with energy', and Roberts (1985) goes on to describe how:

> Very powerful emotions may be evoked: for instance a theme of separation may emerge in a group, evoking powerful responses in each member.

From his experience of art groups, Roberts draws an important distinction between resonance as it develops in verbal group-analytic groups, and how he observed it gathering momentum in art groups: 'Remarkably, while the individuals in a verbal group contribute to "resonance" consecutively, in an art group they contribute concurrently' (Roberts, 1985). This is an important distinction. Visual relating, musical relating and relating through movement in art, dance movement, drama and music therapy groups differs in kind to relating verbally in groups. It is the compound visual–musical–haptic–verbal dimensions and interconnections at play in arts therapies groups which make for a particular kind of group matrix and *embodied* coherence and containment.

Whereas there is a widening understanding of the restorative and transformative qualities of the arts and their role in supporting positive health, health economics look increasingly to evidence from systematic experimental research. Increasingly, evidence for the effectiveness of the arts therapies is becoming available (see Crawford and Patterson, 2007), yet the scaling-up of successful small-scale research pilots to large-scale, multisite randomised control trials has not yet yielded clear benefits (for example, the MATISSE and NESS trials: see Crawford, et al., 2012 and Priebe, et al., 2016 respectively). From research findings, a particular contribution of the arts therapies is seen when working with people with complex traumatisation problems, where experiences cannot be expressed with words because the trauma cannot be thought about in the first place, and where the capacity for making meaningful links is seriously disturbed.

Without recourse here to the audio-visual performance in arts therapies groups, the images, sounds and movements made by individuals and the group-as-a-whole can only be imagined. However, while systematic research in the arts therapies continues, perhaps a quote here by Richard Wollheim (1987) captures something of art's compelling poetry. On the 'imagined sound of time passing' in the paintings of Titian, Wollheim ruminates:

> How does the sound get into these pictures? There is no systematic answer to this question: there is no answer like 'via representation', or 'via expression'. It is rather, as I see it, that the picture gives rise to the thought that the sounds lie around inside it: as we might feel that the notes lie around inside the music box when the tune has stopped, or that the hum lies around inside the fridge. Open up the music box, open up the fridge, open up these paintings, and there we would find the notes. Of course, all these thoughts are metaphorical thoughts, but they are metaphors that record our attempts to capture an impression made upon us. And, once again, these metaphorical thoughts induce the metaphorical thought that they presuppose. The painting is a container: like a body.
>
> (Wollheim, 1987, p. 315)

To understand the poetry at the heart of the arts therapies, more research is required into the mechanisms of change of the arts therapies, and through the microanalysis of the spatio-temporal generative processes operative in arts therapies groups in particular. As one service user said: 'We are changing our minds. We are changing ourselves.'

## Note

1   The collective term 'arts therapies' will be used throughout this chapter to refer to the professional name, recognised in the UK since 1997, for four psychological therapies: art psychotherapy, dance movement psychotherapy, dramatherapy and music therapy.

# References

Crawford, M.J., Killaspy, H., Barnes, T.R.E., Barrett, B., et al. (2012) 'Group art therapy as an adjunctive treatment for people with schizophrenia: Multicentre pragmatic randomised trial'. *British Medical Journal*, 344, e846.

Crawford, M.J. and Patterson, S. (2007) Arts therapies for people with schizophrenia: An emerging evidence base. *Evidence-Based Mental Health*, 10(3), 69–70.

Dratcu, L. (2002) Acute hospital care: The beauty and the beast in psychiatry. *Psychiatric Bulletin*, 26, 81–82.

Foulkes, S.H. (1964) *Therapeutic Group Analysis*. London: George Allen & Unwin.

Gordon, J. and Kirtchuk, G. (2008) *Psychic Assaults and Frightened Clinicians: Countertransference in forensic settings*. London: Karnac Books.

Greenwood, H. (2012) What aspects of an art therapy group aid recovery for people diagnosed with psychosis? *ATOL: Art Therapy Online*, 3(1), 1–32.

Lauschke, M. (2014) 'The bodily communication in picture acts' in S. Marienberg and T. Trabant (Eds), *Bildakt at the Warburg Institute*. Berlin/Boston: Walter de Gruyter.

NICE (National Institute for Health and Care Excellence). (2014) *Psychosis and Schizophrenia in Adults: Prevention and management*. London: NICE.

Nitsun, M. (1996) *The Anti-Group: Destructive forces in the group and their creative potential*. London: Routledge.

Peciccia, M. and Benedetti, G. (1998) The integration of sensorial channels through progressive mirror drawing in the psychotherapy of schizophrenic patients with disturbances in verbal language. *The Journal of the American Academy of Psychoanalysis*, 26(1), 109–122.

Priebe, S., Savill, M., Wykes, T., Bentall, R., et al. (2016) Clinical effectiveness and cost-effectiveness of body psychotherapy in the treatment of negative symptoms of schizophrenia: A multicentre randomised controlled trial. *Health Technology Assessment*, 20(11), vii–xxiii.

Roberts, J.P. (1985) Resonance in art groups. *Inscape*, 1, 17–20.

Roberts, J.P. (1996) 'The importance of Foulke's [*sic*] Matrix Concept'. Retrieved from: www.psychomedia.it/pm/grpther/grpan/robert2a.htm (accessed April 2018).

Rogers, A. (2016) *Incandescent Alphabets: Psychosis and the enigma of language*. London: Karnac Books.

Wollheim, R. (1987) *Painting as an Art*. London: Thames and Hudson.

# Epilogue

## The future of group psychotherapy for psychoses

*Manuel González de Chávez, Ivan Urlić*

In the pages of this book we have witnessed the birth, expansion and consolidation of group therapies in psychoses over an entire century: from the initial reluctances of some professionals, to the progressive acceptance by many others who applied and developed these therapies in their institutions and observed their advantages and therapeutic effects. We have also noted how these group therapies have grown together with other psychotherapies of the psychoses and with the progress of knowledge on groups in general made by sociology and social psychology. In addition, we have observed how the passage from asylum to community psychiatry in the last century has led to the extension and adaptation of group therapies with psychotic patients to numerous organisations and institutions, with the plurality of approaches, perspectives and techniques collected in this book.

Following a century of these therapeutic practices, it is permissible to ask ourselves about the future of group psychotherapies in psychoses. Or even better, we can ask what we should do in the near future to enable a greater number of persons with psychotic experiences to benefit from this therapeutic modality, and what we need to better extend, perfect and adapt it to the needs of these patients.

The existence and development of psychotherapeutic programmes with psychotic patients is a quality indicator of psychiatric care in a country, region or territory, just as the existence of pharmacological monotherapy applied to these patients is an indicator of a low care level. Adequate attention and recovery of persons with psychotic experiences require more complete interventions that will allow them to understand and to overcome their disorders. Today, we can offer them therapeutic help based on many perspectives and modalities from qualified mental health services within a developed and sufficient sociohealth context.

All the therapeutic interventions in persons suffering psychotic disorders are synergic and complementary and should be integrated into flexible care programmes adapted to each patient. We cannot prioritise some of them in detriment to others, nor can we make group therapies the centre of all the care. However, we can procure and promote them in all the organisations that attend persons with these problems, because these group therapies help them to understand and to recover by dynamic means, mechanisms and procedures, and unique and specific therapeutic factors that are presented in different chapters of this book.

In the first decades of the twentieth century, group psychotherapies were no longer measured by cost-effectiveness parameters regarding individual psychotherapies because it soon became clear that the group dynamics of the persons who were parties to the same circumstances and objectives facilitated new disclosures, perspective and motivations, unknown in the dual therapeutic relationship. The meeting in a group therapy context with others having the same or similar disorders and difficulties implies opening a new view of their problems with great therapeutic potential for those persons with psychotic experiences, who take refuge in secrecy, mistrust and isolation. At this time, mental health professionals introduced group therapies with psychotic patients in the most advanced care organisations, as demonstrated in many chapters of this book. This required much dedication, interest and effort to help persons with psychotic experiences in all types of institutions and contexts. This provided better knowledge of these experiences, their possible causes, and pathways to overcoming them. It also gave us better knowledge about the role and work of the group therapists to improve the patient's functionality regarding the therapeutic objectives.

Self-help groups of persons with psychotic disorders came into being in the first decades of the twentieth century. The study of the dynamics and effectiveness of these groups has attracted interest and has had an influence on the future of the group therapies in psychoses. In this book, we have seen that there are hybrid groups, which combine activities or sessions, with and without therapists, and others that are exclusively for persons with psychotic experiences. Included in the latter group are those that consider these experiences with very different conceptual models of disorders; from the traditional medical model, to rejections of any psychopathological consideration of the psychotic experiences, and to the active defence of the normalised redefinition and re-evaluation of them. Among the latter, the Hearing Voices Movement has undergone rapid worldwide expansion, with hundreds of groups in the five continents. This is an indication that the dominant descriptive biological psychiatry is totally insufficient, because it silences more than listens to the patients. There is therefore a need for dynamic psychiatry, with all its psychotherapeutic resources. The growing increase of all the types of self-help groups in the world, especially in countries such as the US, that lack public health services accessible to all the population, is already obligating group therapists to study them more closely. Furthermore, these groups already exist, and 80% of them already count on some type of expert or professional, whether partial or total, regular or irregular, qualified or not qualified, and collaboration or counselling.

Self-help groups have been trying to learn from psychotherapy groups and we, the group therapists, undoubtedly have much to learn from these self-help groups. With groups of psychotic patients and hearers of voices, it is not sufficient to use instructions and declarations of principles or generalisations, or to appeal to a false re-evaluation or normalisation of the psychotic experiences or to voluntarism of self-sufficiencies in the recovery. Psychotic experiences are complex, serious and almost always painful and limiting. No one can ethically predict that professional psychotherapeutic help is perfectly dispensable.

The study of the self-help groups, their creation, development, dynamics, contexts, interactions, leadership, therapeutic factors, influence and results is becoming a growing need and interest for social psychology, sociology and also for the group psychotherapies. However, this same desire should exist in the evaluation procedures of all the group therapies, obviously including psychotherapies with psychotic patients. We need to join care and research, systematically using methodologies based on the practices we perform and not on transient experimental designs that are far from the clinical reality. We should promote and seek the introduction of quality indicators in the usual psychotherapy care, and the systematic and regular study of the variables and most relevant factors. Our field has many uncertainties and a dual complexity, that is, the heterogeneity and the current deficiencies of knowledge of the psychotic experiences, and also the fact that group dynamics are always unique, because the interactions that arise from the grouping and combination of singular and unrepeatable persons are always unique.

With all these difficulties, group psychotherapies in the psychoses have existed for a century, with spectacular advances and developments in all types of institutions and contexts. We have been able to verify this in this book and we hope it will serve for the reflection and training of professionals who are dedicated to group psychotherapy practice. In addition, we hope the book will serve as stimulation for those who want to become involved in the practical learning in therapy groups with psychotic patients. This is because all our groups should be teaching activities and training vehicles that extend these psychotherapies even more, so that a greater number of persons with these experiences that we call psychotic can benefit from them.

Working with our contributors and refining our theoretical stances and practice in applying group work in this specific field concerning psychotic features and personality structures, we believe that we as co-editors were able to express our interest not only in the psychodynamic but in a wide range of cognitive and other approaches. Nowadays we are witnessing the tendency towards 'positive eclecticism' stemming from different clinical experiences and theoretical elaborations. We hope that reading this book will inspire professionals who work with psychotic disturbances to foster their practices and research, and beginners to deepen their interest in internal worlds and meanings of behavioural features of people suffering from psychoses. We do believe in knowledge-based and elaborated creativity.

# Name index

# Subject index